Special Praise for *Dancing in the Dark*

"The set of tools and guidance offered in *Dancing in the Dark* is a valuable resource for the often over-looked caretakers and loved ones of those dealing with depression. The book provides a wealth of information in an engaging and relatable way, which would be beneficial for anyone who has been touched by depression. As a mental health professional who has seen the impact that mental illness has on families, I would highly recommend the tools in this book as a way to navigate the difficult terrain of depression and mental illness."

Kristen M. Anderson
Community Mental Health Worker
Alexandria, Virginia

"A practical guide filled with tools and resources for all those whose lives are touched by depression…written for those just entering 'the dance' as well as those who have been living within the dance for years…written with the sensitivity and understanding that come from experiencing depression first-hand."

Kristine Stache, MA, PhD
Assistant Professor of Missional Leadership
Wartburg Theological Seminary
Dubuque, Iowa

"Living with a significant other who is struggling with depression can be one of life's great challenges. *Dancing in the Dark* provides great insights and practical tools to help you navigate the journey."

Marsha Weaver, MD
Family Medicine Physician
St. Luke's Medical
Overland Park, Kansas

DANCING in the DARK

DANCING in the DARK:

How to Take Care of Yourself When Someone You Love Is Depressed

Bernadette Stankard
Amy Viets

CENTRAL RECOVERY PRESS

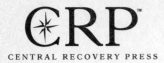

CENTRAL RECOVERY PRESS

Central Recovery Press (CRP) is committed to publishing exceptional materials addressing addiction treatment, recovery, and behavioral health care topics, including original and quality books, audio/visual communications, and web-based new media. Through a diverse selection of titles, we seek to contribute a broad range of unique resources for professionals, recovering individuals and their families, and the general public.

For more information, visit www.centralrecoverypress.com.

Central Recovery Press, Las Vegas, NV 89129

Publisher: Central Recovery Press
          3321 N. Buffalo Drive
          Las Vegas, NV 89129

17 16 15 14 13 12   1 2 3 4 5

ISBN-13: 978-1-936290-70-3 (trade paper)
ISBN-10: 1-936290-70-7 (trade paper)
ISBN-13: 978-1-936290-83-3 (e-book)
ISBN-10: 1-936290-83-9 (e-book)

Bernadette Stankard photo by Edward Stankard
Amy Viets photo by Garrett Viets

Publisher's Note: To protect their privacy, the names of some of the people and institutions in this book have been changed. Central Recovery Press makes no representations or warranties in relation to the medical information in this book; it is not an alternative to medical advice from your doctor or other professional health care provider.

Dancing in the Dark contains general information about depression and suggested treatments. The information is not medical advice, and should not be treated as such. If you have any specific questions about any medical matter you should consult your doctor or other professional health care provider. If you think you or someone close to you may be suffering from any medical condition, including depression, you should seek medical attention promptly. Do not delay seeking medical advice, disregard medical advice, or discontinue medical treatment because of information in this book.

Cover design and interior design and layout by Deb Tremper, Six Penny Graphics

AUTHORS' NOTE

While we are not medical or mental health professionals, our lives have been touched by the pain of depression. If your situation is dire or you fear for your own or your loved one's safety and well-being, contact an emergency room or your doctor immediately.

We are grateful to those who shared their stories with us for the purposes of this book. Their names have been changed to protect their privacy.

Contents

PREFACE

An obituary in the local paper read, "After a gallant fight with depression, Daniel Deavers finally succumbed to suicide. This young father who loved his wife and his children is dead at age thirty-nine." The obituary went on to talk of Daniel's life and his accomplishments and touched briefly on his struggle with depression. Donations to the local mental health association were requested in place of flowers.

Depression had claimed another life. As virulent and elusive as cancer, depression takes lives daily. Many times the illness itself is hidden in death as it often is in life.

People ask, once they learn we write about depression, why we do it. Didn't we have enough of depression when our husbands were themselves suffering from the illness? Don't we want to forget about something that can, well, depress you?

To be truthful, writing about depression is painful. It dredges up memories we would prefer to leave buried. It recalls times we wish we had handled things better. It reminds of us times when we feared our husbands might not survive the illness. But that is only part of the story.

Writing about depression helps us remember that together we overcame a demon that could have devastated us, either physically or emotionally. In the writing, we realized how much we have grown through the experience. We have come to discover happier times together with our spouses, we've moved into a new stage of health and life, and we want to help others do the same.

We had begun to shed light on an issue that had long been ignored: the health and well-being of the caregiver of a depressed person. Comments that have been left on our website, www.depressedspouse.net, show us that we cannot NOT write about depression from the viewpoint of the caregiver.

"I am contacting you because of an 'ah-ha' moment," commented one reader. "I recently purchased your book. I have a clinically depressed spouse and have been struggling with trying to find a way to help him while ignoring myself. I really feel God has blessed me with [your book]. It is wonderful, and it is helping me so much already."

Caregivers have told us that sometimes books are the only avenue they have to give themselves strength. However, few resources are available that are directed solely to the caregiver of a depressed person. We know. We've been there, and we understand the pain expressed in the comments from this reader:

"Your book brought me comfort and helped me see that the illness is what has caused most of this stress for so long. All the other books I've read talk about giving support to your depressed spouse, and, having been on the edge myself, I couldn't do that at times, and therefore those books only increased my guilt. Bless you, as you give hope and comfort to many unsung heroes, who many times suffer alone."

The door we opened in writing our first book about depression is one that many people need opened even wider. In *Dancing in the Dark*, we open the conversation beyond spouses to all the other relationships that are affected by depression. We address postpartum depression, as well as depression in aging relatives, in children, in partners of many loving relationships, and more. Recognizing that depression seeks to destroy anyone in its path, we understand that a whole host of people who love depressed individuals need support and survival skills just as much as the depressed people themselves do.

Depression has claimed enough victims. We cannot and will not allow its darkness to overcome the light of healing and love.

ACKNOWLEDGMENTS

Many people made this book possible. Thanks to Greg Pierce and the people at ACTA Publications, who helped us break ground in the area of support for caregivers of depressed people. We also thank the many people who shared their stories with us, no matter how painful, in the hopes of helping others. Our gratitude also goes to our agent, Jenée Arthur, of the Jenée Arthur Agency, for her expertise, her encouragement, and her sense of humor in the face of such a dark subject. Thanks to Central Recovery Press, for understanding the importance of this book, and to Helen O'Reilly, our editor, and the rest of the CRP staff for their support in getting *Dancing in the Dark* to those who need it. Most especially, we want to thank Ed and Bruce and our children because they keep reminding us how instrumental they are to this book and because they've kept us sane while we revisited those dark days. Working in community makes so many things possible and this book is only one expression of those many possibilities.

CHAPTER ONE

Fighting the Dark

"Dance...wherever you may be."

Sydney Carter[*]

Dancing has long been an artistic form of expression. Hip-hop and square dancing, tango and salsa—we are caught up in the beauty of the movement and the grace of the dancers. Dancing moves our bodies as well as our souls, helping us to celebrate. We often forget, however, that dancing with our feet is not the only way to dance.

The dance steps you will find in this book call you to dance with the heart— they can be seen in the welcome of a spouse after a year overseas or in the birth of a baby into a family. They can be seen even in the darkest of times, at a dying person's bedside or an unexpected funeral. The dance is done by a heart overflowing with joy, gratitude, sorrow, or hope. This dancing takes more than limbs, more than grace and beauty. It takes an attitude of openness, and a willingness to try the new steps no matter how taxing and painful they might be.

---

[*]   From "Lord of the Dance" by Sydney Carter, © 1963 Stainer & Bell, Ltd. (Hope Publishing Company, Carol Stream, IL 60188). All rights reserved. Used by permission.

Meditation

"The heart is like a garden. It can grow
compassion or fear, resentment or love.
What seeds will you plant there?"

The Buddha

Many of us are comfortable living with the weeds that have grown in our hearts—the resentments, the "I don't care" attitudes, the wounded stances. Just as it takes hard work to pull weeds out of the flower garden, it takes work to cultivate a good attitude, to look squarely at those resentments and do something about them, to acknowledge the pain and do something about it. Sometimes it is too much hard work, but just as with the garden full of weeds, our hearts respond to our beginning steps to do something, our beginning steps to dance. One weed pulled is one weed fewer. One move toward a positive response is one step closer.

Help me make the decision to begin to
weed the garden of my heart.

Depression is an odd place to find a dance in progress. It is an odd place to dance and to rejoice. However, unless we learn to dance during depression, we, as well as our loved ones, can be swallowed by the dark. When depression darkens our lives, the dance steps might be far from us. Our hearts may feel stilled and unable to dance. It is vital, however, that we find the form of dance that is right for us, the dance that will dispel the darkness and move us toward recovery.

Depression itself takes many forms. One person with depression sleeps all day. One yells at the kids. Another cries uncontrollably. Still another might face a monumental task in deciding what pair of socks to wear.

Depression Statistics

- Major depressive disorder is the leading cause of disability in the United States for ages fifteen through forty-four.

- Major depressive disorder affects approximately 14.8 million American adults, or about 6.7 percent of the US population age eighteen and older in a given year.

- While major depressive disorder can develop at any age, the median age at onset is thirty-two.

- Major depressive disorder is more prevalent in women than in men.

National Institute of Mental Health[1]

Having lived with depressed people ourselves, we know how difficult the illness can be for them. We also know self-care is not a simple task when you are worn out with caring for someone else. Looking back, both of us wish there had been dance lessons available to us, tools that would have taught our souls to dance during our partners' depression. We did stumble across some ideas of our own along the way, and we discovered more coping strategies as we talked with others about how they survived depression in a loved one.

Experience with Depression

Amy's Journey

My husband's depression had, we now realize, been present most of his life. It wasn't until we were married and had our first child that the illness became too great for him to hide it. He went into a long, slow tailspin, which came to a head in both physical and emotional crises. Then came the seemingly endless parade of tests, doctors, therapists, drugs, and diagnoses. There were twelve years in which no relief was in sight, and the darkness that shrouded my husband daily encroached on my own soul as well. I lost connection with my God, I lost connection with my husband, and I lost connection with any form of joyous dancing in my own heart.

I was and am thankful that there were points of light I could cling to along the way. Motherhood was a calling that fed my soul even in the worst of times. There were friends who empathized, offered support, and helped me laugh. Still, there were many tearful days and nights, much emptiness and fear and despair.

It was only in hindsight, when we finally found healing and recovery, that I began to recognize things I did during the struggle with depression that helped dispel the darkness. Once the pain was a distant memory, I took a look at what I might have done differently, tools I might have employed, in order to nurture the dance in my heart.

Bernadette's Journey

Having finally come to terms with my addiction to alcohol, I thought we were, as a couple and a family, ready for some smoother sailing. How wrong I was! Ed's depression had been present in his life from the time of his father's death when Ed was only five, and it moved to full-blown major depression during our married years. There were panic attacks and unpredictable moods, too much sleep, and irritability. With two young children, sometimes I found myself at wit's end, with no family to turn to, few friends who really understood, and a Higher Power who seemed to be too busy helping all the other people in twelve-step programs.

Without my knowledge, my Higher Power, whom I'd thought too busy, was also working for me, teaching me dance steps at a rate I could handle. Looking back, I can clearly see instances of my Higher Power at work— sending me a friend when I needed companionship, a listening ear when things got really difficult, a babysitter when I needed to get away, the right medication for Ed when there was no other place to turn. My Higher Power, whom I call God, was helping me to dance with Ed on the road to recovery.

Reflections

- *If you needed to tell your story to someone, who would that be? In whom do you have enough trust to share your story?*

- *What are some painful points of your story?*

- *What positive points do you see?*

....

Now that we and our partners have emerged on the other side of depression, we recognize how important it is to share these tools with others. We know growing and remaining healthy is possible despite the darkness of the illness, and we believe the tools we offer in these pages can help make a time of depression become a time of self-awareness rather than a time of misery and stagnation.

Because depression isn't the same for everyone, those who care for depressed people must use a number of strategies to survive a period of depression in a loved one. Therefore, this book offers a variety of tools, including meditations and related actions and exercises. Choose the ones that are right for you, that help you and your loved one grow through the darkness of depression and dance to the light on the other side.

Making a PACT

A pact, or a commitment, calls us to be intentional and faithful in relationship. As a basis for the tools we offer, we use an acronym, PACT, which reminds us of the need for relationship with our Higher Power and with others. The intentional use of the four components of PACT can help us survive the depression of a loved one.

A **PACT** to survive the depression of a loved one:

Prayer

Affirmation

Community

Truth

PRAYER

Prayer means different things to different people, but after all is said and done, it is simply a time of conversation and relationship with our Higher Power, celebrating gifts, asking for help, and laughing and crying together. Prayer helps us gather strength from our Higher Power, through whatever channel that power manifests itself. Maintaining a relationship with our Higher Power, whoever or whatever the Higher Power is, especially during painful times in our lives, can make it possible for us to continue when we're afraid all is lost. Many who have been able to stay connected to their Higher Power through hard times have discovered a surprising strength and peace coming from that relationship. Tools to help you develop your relationship with your Higher Power are necessary to your survival, and are an important part of this book.

AFFIRMATION

Affirmation is a stream of goodness flowing into our lives and the lives of others. When depression intrudes on a relationship, words and acts of affirmation often disappear. Living with someone who exhibits the typical symptoms of depression, such as lack of energy, irritability, and anger, can take a toll on the nondepressed person's self-confidence and self-esteem. Learning how to remind ourselves of our own value, and the value in which our Higher Power holds us, and learning to be open to receiving affirmation from others in our lives can enable us to remember not only the beauty in ourselves but also the beauty in our loved one.

COMMUNITY

There's no way around it—we need people. In good times, we want family and friends around us to share our joy. When times are bad, we need our community even more if we are to get through with our souls intact. Community helps us with prayer, with meals and practical assistance, with hugs and supportive words. Community uplifts us when depression starts to pull us down. Community, and recognizing the presence of our Higher Power within it, can allow us to be open to this love and support, which we need for staying whole.

TRUTH

When, in the midst of depression, we hold our pain close to us, refusing to share with those who are worthy of trust, the pain grows and takes on monstrous proportions. Pain and fear grow in darkness. Truth, on the other hand, is the light of day. Sharing the truth of our pain and fear, when we know what to share and whom to share it with, is like the sun coming out after a storm. We must learn to drop our facades—with ourselves, our loved ones, and others—if we are to remain healthy and whole.

> "There is a people sent from God whose name is Hope.
> And the people named Hope shall bear witness to the light;
> Despair shall not overcome us.
> There is a people sent from God whose name is Love.
> And the people named Love shall bear witness to the light;
> Hatred shall not overwhelm us.
> There is a people sent from God whose name is Life.
> And the people named Life shall bear witness to the light;
> Death shall not overpower us." [2]

Depression is an equal-opportunity destroyer. It destroys the lives of countless men and women as they struggle with an illness that takes away joy. For those living with a depressed person, the use of PACT and the tools offered in this book can make the difference between night and day. Whatever the outcome of our loved one's depression, if we learn to dance, using the steps that are right for us and practicing them with regularity, we can move through this hard time. We can come out healthier and happier despite our encounter with the darkness called depression.

> "Can I see another's woe, and not be in sorrow too? Can I
> see another's grief, and not seek for kind relief?"
>
> William Blake

The illness called depression is painful to watch. When it attacks someone for whom we care deeply, we, too, are affected. Whatever our reaction— whether we withdraw in fear or reach out to comfort and assist—we are forever changed by the close-up view of the intense suffering of another.

Through the experience of stepping in as caregivers to husbands diagnosed with clinical depression, we have learned the pitfalls and joys of coming through this darkness with the ability to dance. It is our hope that you find some strength and guidance as you, too, attempt to navigate the darkness of depression. If your situation is dire, or you fear for your own or your loved one's safety and well-being, contact an emergency room or your doctor immediately.

The appendix of *Dancing in the Dark* provides prompts and suggestions you can use to reflect on any thoughts or ideas in the book that speak to you. You can refer to this section as you read. We suggest you read with a highlighter, pen, or sticky notes in order to mark items you wish to return to as you continue your journey with a depressed loved one. We invite you to use a separate journal to complete any suggested exercises that require extra space.

CHAPTER ONE NOTES

1. National Institute of Mental Health. 2010. *Major Depressive Disorder Among Adults* [Online]. Available from http://www.nimh.nih.gov/statistics/1MDD_ADULT.shtml (accessed 8 August 2010).

2. *Litanies and Other Prayers for the Revised Common Lectionary Year B*, Phyllis Cole and Everett Tilson (Nashville, Abingdon Press, 1993.) Used by permission. All rights reserved.

CHAPTER TWO

The Darkness Knocks at the Door

"When it is dark enough, you can see the stars."

Ralph Waldo Emerson

D epression may come as suddenly as a light being switched off in a room or as quietly as the dark rolling in after a brilliant sunset. It may come swiftly, like nightfall after a long summer day. Or it may just be there, like a long, gloomy day with sudden violent storms punctuating the bleakness.

Depression can bring with it overflowing emotion or none at all. It brings questions and frustrations, second-guessing and fear, helplessness and anger. For the sufferer it brings a self-loathing, a loss of the spirit that can affect work and love and even the very reason for living. Deep, abiding depression can affect relationships between the depressed person and those who love him or her. It can cut deeply into how the person thinks of him- or herself, opening the door to self-destruction in many forms.

When we watch depression grow in someone we love, we too are affected in our spirits. Often our self-esteem plummets and our ability to care for ourselves and others is severely impaired. It is only when we recognize and act on the depression affecting our relationships that we are able to make a difference both in our own well-being and in that of our depressed loved one. However, taking action is no easy task.

Depression does not always have standard, easily recognizable symptoms that are consistent from one person to another. There might be extra sleeping, or lack of sleep; bouts of sadness, or angry outbursts. Increased irritability might indicate something is wrong. We might become aware of feelings of guilt or worthlessness in the depressed person. Appetite might swing to overeating or undereating. However depression expresses itself in the early stages, it is important for the well-being of everyone involved to become aware and be ready to address the challenge in a measured way. It is our loving care and intervention that spells the difference between the depressed person seeking help and falling deeper into the dark pit. That intervention might also be the thing that saves our own quality of life.

Meditation

"Tonight we reflect on paradox; Water wears away rock. Spirit overcomes force. The weak will undo the mighty. May we learn to see things backwards, inside out, and upside down."

Adapted from the *Tao Te Ching*

The story is told of a deep puddle under a tree, close to a river. Day after day the few fish in the puddle would swim around in circles, fighting each other for water bugs. One day a beautiful rainbow fish dropped into the puddle. He talked of jumping from the puddle into the river and being carried to the ocean because the ocean was where fish were meant to be. All the fish shook their heads in sadness and distress and stubbornness, except for one fish who nervously said he would jump with the rainbow fish and see this glorious ocean. Those two fish jumped from

the puddle and into the river and were carried to the
ocean, the place they were meant to be, which was filled
with wonders beyond imagination. The other fish? They
continued to swim in circles, fighting for water bugs.

When depression strikes our lives, we have two courses
of action: stay in the puddle and swim aimlessly or take
the leap into new ways of acting, new ways, as the *Tao Te
Ching* says, of seeing things—backwards, inside out, and
upside down.

> *Lord, today help me to keep a positive,*
> *fresh outlook on everything.*

The First Line of Defense

Depression affects not only the sufferer but also those who touch the
depressed person's life. A clear understanding of what depression is and how
it affects each and every player is our best and first line of defense.

According to annual estimates, over 18.8 million American adults suffer
from some sort of depression. Sadly, most do not seek help. But those who
do seek help very often experience improvement. Why, then, don't more
depressed individuals request help? Often, they cannot come to terms with
their illness, or there is no one available to help them navigate the steep
slope to recovery. Depression itself often makes it too difficult to take the
action necessary to obtain help.

Depression is an illness involving the whole body, according to the National
Institute of Mental Health. It can affect how we feel physically, mentally,
emotionally, and spiritually. A depressed person may complain of physical
aches and pains. He or she may shout or react violently, when in the past
there was only gentleness. If the depressed person is someone we care about

deeply, we feel the sting of rejection when he or she is no longer able to express that love. We may feel abandoned when our Higher Power doesn't seem to hear our pleas for the one we love.

Although there are many ways depression manifests itself, there are two common types of depression.

Major depression is an illness that interferes with daily life. An overwhelming feeling of sadness is present, along with lack of interest in things that formerly were important. No longer is the individual able to perform routine daily activities at home or work. Appetite and sleep can be affected. A person suffering from major depression will often have several of the symptoms of depression. (See sidebar, page 15.)

Dysthymia (dis-THIGH-mee-*uh)* is a milder form of depression. Sometimes referred to as lifelong depression, dysthymia is long-term and chronic but doesn't necessarily affect day-to-day interactions. The list of symptoms for dysthymia is the same as for major depression, but symptoms are usually less severe. However, it is common for dysthymia to develop into major depression. Many of those suffering from dysthymia often have difficulty functioning at full capacity and/or feel chronically unwell. A person suffering from dysthymia is unlikely to be able to celebrate the joys of life as a normally functioning individual can.

What causes depression? There are various factors, according to researchers. Some types of depression run in families. Depression triggered by major life events that create stress is often referred to as situational depression. Job loss and depression often go hand in hand. Biochemical imbalances in the brain certainly play a role. Certain physical illnesses such as cancer, stroke, diabetes, heart disease, and HIV/AIDS can change a person's brain chemistry, leading to depression. No matter the causes or triggers, a variety of factors can contribute to this illness, impairing a person's ability to live life to its fullest. Depression is also a factor in some suicides.

Depression Statistics

- In focus groups created to assess depression awareness, men described their own symptoms of depression without realizing that they were depressed.

National Institute of Mental Health, 2008[1]

- Women experience twice the rate of depression as men, regardless of race or ethnic background.

National Alliance on Mental Illness, 2010[2]

- Although black Americans are less likely than whites to have a major depressive disorder (MDD), when they do it tends to be more chronic and severe. They are also much less likely to undergo treatment.

National Institute of Mental Health, 2007[3]

- Depression affects more than 6.5 million of the 35 million Americans aged sixty-five years or older.

National Alliance on Mental Illness, 2010[4]

- Numerous studies reveal that most suicide attempts by homosexuals occur during their youth. Gay youth are two to three times more likely to attempt suicide than other young people.

Getting Help

Mark sleeps late every day. Very late. On weekdays his partner, Rob, does his best to ignore it. After all, Mark isn't working and doesn't have a job to get to. Rob, on the other hand, has a half-hour commute to work and needs to be on his way by 7:15 every morning. So he goes about his daily routine and heads out the door with a last glance at the bedroom, where he knows Mark will be in bed for most of the morning—maybe even most of the day.

On the subway, Rob does his best to downplay in his mind what's happening at home. He has a good job, one that pays enough to allow Mark to stay at home during the day. It doesn't matter that he sleeps so much. Really, it doesn't. Right? So why does Rob find his jaw clenched so tightly every morning that it makes his head hurt? Why this burning frustration churning in his stomach as he nears home each evening? Why is it that lately a few of his coworkers have commented that his mind seems to be elsewhere?

Rob doesn't realize it yet, but he's dealing with the fallout from depression.

Reflections

- *What is my situation like? What similarities do I notice between Rob's story and my own?*

- *What is especially bothering me regarding my loved one? What particular symptom is present?*

- *What changes have I noticed in myself since all this started with my loved one?*

When we live with a person whose habits, behavior, and emotions slide into a descent, it takes some time to recognize just how bad things have gotten. If we don't have prior experience or knowledge about the illness called depression, it can take even longer. It's hard to name something when we don't know much about it. Even when we are informed about common symptoms of depression, the stigma that has long been attached to such mental illnesses makes it difficult to accept reality, or the prospect of dealing with such an illness seems so overwhelming that we try to ignore what's right in front of us.

Depressed or Just "Down"?

So what is depression, exactly? Certainly it is a medical condition that can be treated, often with medications, psychotherapy, or other methods. It may involve a genetic chemical imbalance, or it may be situational, involving life circumstances. Whatever the cause, unlike many physical illnesses, there is no simple test for diagnosing depression. Instead, diagnosis depends on assessment by a professional, based on reported behaviors and feelings. Herein lies the conundrum: those who are suffering from depression may be unable to articulate their own behaviors and feelings, or they may recognize that they feel rotten but don't have the energy to face that fact and seek help.

Symptoms of Depression

- Feelings of sadness or unhappiness

- Irritability or frustration, even over small matters

- Loss of interest or pleasure in normal activities

- Reduced sex drive

- Insomnia or excessive sleeping

- Changes in appetite—depression often causes decreased appetite and weight loss, but in some people it causes increased cravings for food and weight gain

- Agitation or restlessness—for example, pacing, hand-wringing, or an inability to sit still

- Slowed thinking, speaking, or body movements

- Indecisiveness, distractibility, and decreased concentration

- Fatigue, tiredness, and loss of energy—even small tasks may seem to require a lot of effort

- Feelings of worthlessness or guilt, fixating on past failures, or blaming yourself when things aren't going right

- Trouble thinking, concentrating, making decisions, and remembering things

- Frequent thoughts of death, dying, or suicide

- Crying spells for no apparent reason

- Unexplained physical problems, such as back pain or headaches

Mayo Clinic, 2010[5]

It often falls to a loved one to make the call. Is this person I care about just going through a "down" period, or is he or she actually clinically depressed? Here again, there can be some problems inherent in trying to make that call. We can be reluctant to admit a serious problem is present, for a number of reasons. Sometimes we are too close to the situation to see it clearly for what it is. Mental illness makes many people uncomfortable, and often we feel ill-equipped to deal with such a major illness. There might be some idea of what's involved in seeking help and finding treatment, but we still feel overwhelmed by the prospect. It's easier to look the other way and hope things will improve without our help.

But at some point, it becomes clear things will not improve on their own. Our own frustration level, our concern for our loved one, the effects ongoing depression can have on our lives, eventually bring the situation to a head. Dealing with the problem, at some point, becomes inevitable.

There is a rule of thumb that can help us make the call between possible depression and just a "down" period. It's generally recognized that if at least five common symptoms of depression are present consistently for two weeks, further investigation and treatment of some sort are probably needed.

Physical factors other than depression can create similar symptoms. Diabetes, thyroid problems, and many other illnesses can be a possibility.

It is in everyone's best interest to get the affected person to a health professional to address the root causes of the behaviors that are so upsetting. A good place to start determining what is happening is with a good physical examination. If that examination shows nothing else is causing the symptoms, it is time to move on to a mental health professional for diagnosis and treatment.

Why Do I Have to Be the One to Deal with This?

We tend to operate on the assumption that as adults, we are responsible for taking care of ourselves. If the heater in the car is on the fritz, we take the car in to the mechanic. If we have a sinus infection, we see a doctor and get any needed antibiotics. Generally, we don't need the assistance of friends, family, spouses, or partners to handle these things. Sure, we ask for their advice, but on the whole we can handle things on our own. Those of us listening to a friend, family member, spouse, or partner will have a sympathetic ear and true caring, but such issues often don't have a major impact on our own day-to-day functioning.

An intimate partner's or family member's depression, on the other hand, is not something we can just "work around." Depending on the degree of closeness between the depressed person and ourselves, depression has the potential to have a profound impact on our daily lives. Depression brings with it a heavy cloud of negative thoughts, feelings, and behaviors. Depressed people can snarl with irritation over something we would normally expect them to shrug off. They can be easily confused, leading to misunderstandings. They may have trouble making decisions, holding you in a conversation about what outfit to wear long after you're dressed and ready to walk out the door. In short, many behaviors associated with depression have direct, negative, and frustrating consequences for innocent but concerned friends, family, and loved ones.

Try This

Pull out a picture of your loved one and paste it to the middle of a sheet of paper. On a separate sheet, in the middle of the paper, write the word **DEPRESSION**. On the first sheet, around your loved one's picture, write all the words you can think of that were and are positive about him or her, or write of instances when you particularly appreciated him or her. On the second sheet, around the word **DEPRESSION**, write all the words of anger and sadness that fill you when you encounter depression in your loved one. This exercise will help you remember that your parent or partner or child or friend does not equal depression; rather, depression is a force that can and does eat away at both of you if you let it.

Any time someone we love shows signs of a serious illness, we want to step in with help and support, in the best interests of our loved one. When the serious illness is depression, stepping in is vital, both for our own self-preservation and for that of our depressed loved one. If we let the situation continue unabated, the frustration we feel in dealing with the depressed person can easily turn into anger. Sometimes the depressed person is someone we've come to count on as a life partner. In this case, we can be left without assistance in the everyday aspects of life, from financial decision-making to child rearing. Handling everything alone, while also dealing with the unpleasant symptoms of depression, can cause us to head into a downward spiral ourselves. It's worth it, even if only for our own health and sanity, to help a loved one who may be depressed seek treatment.

Meditation

*"Be patient toward all that is unsolved in
your heart and try to love the questions
themselves, like locked rooms and like books
that are written in a very foreign tongue."*

Rainer Maria Rilke

"Why is the sky blue?"

"Why do people have two legs and dogs have four legs?"

"Why is it light in the daytime and dark in the night?"

This is typical conversation for a four-year-old. "Why"
questions are a young child's way of trying to make sense
of the world, trying to put life into order.

When depression intrudes on a cherished relationship,
"why" questions bombard us from all directions. "Why
is this happening to my loved one?" "Why is this illness
affecting me, too?" "Why doesn't my Higher Power hear
my cries of fear, of despair, of anger?" In the midst of
confusion and hurt, these questions are our way of trying
to make sense of it all.

Keeping Rilke's words in mind, we can cultivate patience
for these unsolved questions. We can continue to cry out
to our Higher Power—that Power is listening and caring,
whether we can believe it or not—and accept that these
questions are a part of life. Like books in a foreign tongue,
we may not understand them now; but with patience, with
practice, with time, our Higher Power can guide us to
healing and eventual understanding.

God, help me understand and accept the "whys" of life.

Dealing with Anger

The illness of depression in a loved one can bring out strong emotions in the nondepressed person in the relationship. If not addressed, the frustration, the wondering "why us?" manifests itself in surprising ways, including anger. Anger wears many faces. It's easy to recognize anger that is open and direct, but the anger that lurks beneath the surface is tricky. We may find ourselves being sarcastic with our loved one, or we may find ourselves withdrawing from situations we previously enjoyed. We sometimes resort to passive-aggressive behavior, in which we know exactly what our depressed loved one wants and needs but we simply do not provide it. Blaming, being critical, or just being too exhausted to care could all be ways of expressing anger.

One of the most important things for someone living with a depressed person to do is to acknowledge his or her anger and try to give it over to the Higher Power. This is certainly difficult to do, as we humans like to hold onto our angry feelings. After all, we have been wounded, we have been hurt. Depression has been described by some as "anger turned inward." Unless we attempt to let go of overwhelming anger about the situation or toward our loved one, we could fall victim to depression as well.

Recognizing Anger

Common symptoms of anger include:

- Increased heart rate

- Shallow breathing

- Tense muscles; for example, clenched jaws or fists

- Single-minded focus on or obsession with an upsetting issue

- Difficulty looking at or smiling at the person with whom you feel angry

- Words that fly out without thought or filter

Of course, each of us displays anger differently. Over the course of a week or so, pay attention to your own feelings and actions so you can recognize your specific symptoms.

Chasing the Anger Away

When dealing with the anger caused by depression, we first must acknowledge that it is present. "Nice" people don't feel anger, we may think. Actually, anger is a human emotion, neither bad nor good in itself. It is in the expression of anger that problems arise—and one all-too-common reaction of many people, whether dealing with depression or not, is refusing to be aware of their own anger. Ignoring anger can lead to expressions of anger that are hurtful, dismaying, and frightening, to ourselves as much as to those around us. When we acknowledge we are grappling with angry feelings—of feeling abandoned, of wanting to lash out, of wondering "Why me?"—healing can begin.

We can start with simple actions. A mantra to remind ourselves that the anger *just is* may be helpful. "I'm angry at the disease, not the person." "I am angry that my loved one is suffering." "I am angry at this feeling of helplessness." These types of inwardly directed comments can be helpful in acknowledging the anger and moving beyond it.

When anger creeps into your heart, try to pause and consider what is really taking place. Acknowledge that you are dealing with an individual who is grappling with a debilitating disease. Take a deep breath, breathing from your core. Let the breath out slowly, thinking to yourself, "This too shall pass." Try to look at the situation as a bystander. What would that bystander do if he or she were in your place? How would he or she talk to your loved one?

Go beyond simply acknowledging the anger, and remind yourself that anger is a reasonable reaction to an unreasonable situation. Find ways to release energy when that energy is the negative type associated with anger. Exercise, escape through a good book or movie, do an activity like weeding the garden. These deliberate distractions or escapes turn the negative energy into something positive. When you're able to make this shift, a sense of accomplishment and pride can replace a sense of despair and frustration.

Too often we fall into repetitive, negative patterns in dealing with those we love. We forget to truly listen, to try to hear what they are saying as if for the first time. Deliberately concentrating on accepting and mastering our anger can help to temper it and bring the whole situation into perspective. Accept and embrace the good as well as the not-so-good. Dance in the dark. It can make all the difference.

Peace and the Healing Process

One of the great maxims of twelve-step recovery worldwide is "Let go and let God." Following this advice frees up a great deal of energy we use fighting our loved one, fighting the depression, fighting our own responses, and it lets our Higher Power enter our lives. By giving ourselves over to the guidance and love of our Higher Power, we are able to concentrate on what needs to be done so healing can happen. When we calm our own minds in this way, we may be more able or willing to respond to the needs we see before us—both for our loved ones and for ourselves.

Our situation can't change if we don't make changes. We can't rely on the same patterns of behavior we used when our loved one was well. Change in our attitude, in our responses, and in our relationship with our Higher Power and with others will enable us to make the changes necessary for dealing with this dark illness. Doctor's appointments will be made, dinners cooked and eaten, arguments averted with positive action. All these things will happen if we allow change to happen.

Some of us can do this naturally; for others it takes practice. To do anything well takes practice and perseverance; so it is with dancing. If we are to dance in the dark with the one who is suffering from depression, we have to acknowledge that life is not always what we want it to be. We need to make the best of it because that is the only way to be happy. Practice acknowledging that depression is not what we would want for ourselves or our loved one. Practice making the best of the situation, even if—especially if—that means squeezing in some quiet time for ourselves. Continually carrying all the anger, all the worry, all the frustration will only cause our load to become heavier and more difficult to handle. Trusting in our Higher Power to handle the worries and frustrations is the only way we will remain healthy and able to dance toward recovery.

"The feeling remains that God is on the journey, too."

St. Teresa of Avila

CHAPTER TWO NOTES

1. National Institute of Mental Health. 2008. *Men and Depression* [Online]. Available from http://www.nimh.nih.gov/health/publications/men-and-depression/complete-index.SHTML (accessed 21 July 2010).

2. National Alliance on Mental Illness. 2010. *Women and Depression* [Online]. Available from http://www.nami.org/template.cfm?section=depression (accessed 21 July 2010).

3. National Institute of Mental Health. 2007. *African Americans, Black Caribbeans, and Whites Differ in Depression Risk, Treatment* [Online]. Available from http://www.nimh.nih.gov/science-news/2007/african-americans-black-caribbeans-and-whites-differ-in-depression-risk-treatment.shtml (accessed 21 July 2010).

4. National Alliance on Mental Illness. 2010. *Depression in Older Persons Fact Sheet* [Online]. Available from http://www.nami.org/Template.cfm?Section=By_Illness&template=/ContentManagement/ContentDisplay.cfm&ContentID=7515 (accessed 21 July 2010).

5. Mayo Clinic. 2010. *Depression (major depression)* [Online]. Available from http://www.mayoclinic.com/health/depression/DS00175/DSECTION=symptoms (accessed 8 July 2010).

CHAPTER THREE

Finding Your Way in the Dark

"Each player must accept the cards life deals him or her: but once they are in hand, he or she alone must decide how to play the cards in order to win the game."

Voltaire

When you play a game of gin, you're dealt a hand of seven cards. The rules of the game state that you must always keep seven cards in your hand, but you can choose new and, it is to be hoped, better cards, as long as you let go of a card you already hold in place of each new card you choose. It's a difficult decision, choosing new cards, considering the risks involved in keeping or trading. Always, the goal is a winning hand.

And so goes the process of discerning the correct treatment for depression. There are guidelines for how to play, and the ever-present variables of new treatments, new doctors, new therapists. We wonder whether the course we have in hand is the best combination. We wonder if there are other possibilities out there that could better help us reach our goal, but we worry about the risk of discarding what's in hand for something new.

Thanks to research, new medications, and increasing awareness, the illness of depression is treatable. The medical community recognizes that a combination of antidepressant medication and psychotherapy creates the best opportunity for relief from depression symptoms. Sounds like a fairly simple recipe, right? Take a pill every day, visit a therapist every week or two, and things will get better soon. Unfortunately, effective depression treatment is a lot more difficult than that. There are a lot more steps to recovery, and even though we know the steps to take, the correct steps too often seem hidden. It's very easy to miss them in the dark and take a painful tumble.

Medication

There are several classes of antidepressants, each with its own benefits and hazards. Within these classes are various dosages and subtle differences. Any antidepressant takes at least two to three weeks to reach effectiveness. Along with this time of waiting in hope for the medicine to make a positive difference, there's the need to watch for negative side effects. Side effects vary widely, and can be difficult to differentiate from the effects of depression itself. After a two- to three-week period, there's the need to evaluate just how much improvement—if any—is noted. The depressed person is often unable to judge improvement realistically, requiring the input of someone who can observe changes for the better or worse. This process means repeated visits to a psychopharmacologist, a doctor who specializes in the treatment of depression with medication, who may or may not be able to see the depressed person within a reasonable time frame.

But that's only one aspect of the treatment equation. Psychotherapy is an equally important factor. With the assistance of a therapist, behaviors can be changed to facilitate relief from depression. Hurts from the past, mishandled anger, painful issues that have contributed to depression can be uncovered and dealt with, helping the depressed person move on with new ways to cope.

Psychotherapy can present its own difficulties, however. Sadly, health insurers have not kept pace with the rest of us in recognizing the fundamental importance of treating depression to maintain health; therapy for depression and other mental illnesses is rarely covered adequately by insurance. Finding the right therapist to work with is a hurdle, as well. Just as there are some people we wouldn't choose as close friends, there are some people who aren't a good fit in therapy. How and when does the depressed person decide to try someone new? Where does he or she even go to find another person who might be a better fit? How long will it take to get an appointment? How accessible is the new therapist's schedule? The hand we're dealt in this high-stakes game can be difficult and confusing.

Depression Treatment Statistics

- Despite the availability of treatment for depression, only 39 percent of people with severe depression reported contacting a mental health professional in the past year.

- Of 2.4 billion drugs prescribed in visits to doctors and hospitals in 2005, 118 million were for antidepressants.

U.S. Centers for Disease Control and Prevention, 2005[1]

- Antidepressants ranked as the leading therapy class by dispensed prescription volume in 2007.

IMS Health Reports[2]

- The Substance Abuse and Mental Health Services Administration found that 71 percent of adults who had major depression used mental health services and treatment to help with their disorder. Generally, women and adults over fifty were more likely than men and younger adults to use services for depression.

National Survey on Drug Use and Health, 2008[3]

Making the Decision to Step In

It's a cruelly ironic aspect of depression that just when a person most needs to reach out for help, he or she is most unable to do so. Fatigue, despair, and other symptoms of depression keep many depressed people from seeking and/or following through with treatment. Sometimes the only thing making treatment and recovery possible is the presence of someone in the depressed person's life who is willing to step in and help navigate the maze of doctors, medications, and therapy.

When we observe the darkness of depression descending upon someone we care about, we have questions to ask ourselves: At what point—if any—do I offer my help? Am I qualified to assist in this situation? Are the person and I close enough? Do I know anything about depression treatment? Do I have the time and the energy to become part of this process? Questioning and indecision are common reactions to this situation. But decisions must be made.

In some relationships, the answers are clear and obvious. In others, the degree of involvement is less clear-cut, and it takes a great deal of thoughtful reflection to come to a decision. As with so many situations in life, our action is often spurred when we realize we can no longer NOT "do something." For those who are unfamiliar with the ins and outs of depression treatment, getting involved as a facilitator in the recovery process is a daunting prospect. We need to be honest with ourselves about what we feel capable of doing, and exactly what our standing is.

Reflections

- *What is the history of my relationship with the depressed person about whom I'm concerned?*

- *Where do I stand currently with this person?*

- *What level of intervention am I able to provide? How much time and energy can I offer?*

- *What do I know about treatment for depression? Am I willing and able to learn what we need to know in order to help him or her find relief?*

- *Is there anyone else close to this person who might be able to be of assistance during this time?*

....

Offering Help

Once you've clarified in your own mind your role in your loved one's recovery, it's necessary to discuss the subject with the person of concern. This conversation, though, can be more difficult than it sounds. Offering help for depression means naming the problem and addressing it. Admitting the presence of depression can be a serious obstacle. Those of us who have experience with what depression can do to people are thankful that what was once a forbidden subject is becoming an acceptable topic of conversation. However, though we've made great progress in our society in destigmatizing the illness, many people still consider depression to be a sign of weakness, shameful and embarrassing. The depth of depression, too, is a concern. The depressed person's ability to talk about the subject might be seriously affected.

Therefore, it's necessary to consider what the person's feelings and preconceptions might be about the illness of depression. It's also important to ask yourself how far down the road to depression he or she seems to be. Consider what you've noticed recently concerning your loved one's ability to discuss serious topics. If the question of possible depression has come up in the past, think about what his or her reaction was at that time.

When you're ready for a conversation, choose the time carefully. Look for a window of opportunity, if there is one, when your loved one is more "up"— perhaps after a relaxing activity, and when he or she is well rested. Choose your words carefully as well. Though you'll probably need to describe the changes in behavior and mood you've noticed, avoid any hint of accusation or derision. Even though these behavior and mood changes are likely to have been hard on you, work to keep anger and hurt out of your tone. Save your need for an emotional dump—and it's certainly a legitimate need—for someone outside this situation.

Reassure the depressed person of your love and your commitment to helping him or her feel like him- or herself again. Gauge carefully the reaction you receive as you decide how far to carry the conversation. There's every chance that your offer will need some time to sink in. Don't feel like specific treatment decisions need to be made right away. If necessary, drop the conversation and come back to it as soon as is reasonably possible. Just as persistence in the face of the medication and therapy challenges is the key to successful treatment, persistence in discussing the problem with your loved one is sometimes required.

It's hard to admit when one wants so much to help, but the right person to help our loved one might be someone other than ourselves. We may be too close to the situation, or perhaps we are not close enough to bring up such a delicate topic. Maybe we know that to do so would cause more harm. Perhaps we feel uncomfortable ourselves with the topic of depression. In these cases, turn to a professional for help and suggestions. In any event, doing something is necessary for the sake of the depressed person and for the people who live close to the disease.

Resistance to Treatment

But what if your loved one reacts poorly? What if he or she refuses to accept the possibility of depression, refuses to see a doctor, refuses to consider looking into any type of treatment? It can happen. Whether due to fear of stigma, intimidation at the very thought of tackling the problem, or other factors, some people will reject the idea of seeking treatment. Some will even become angry and react harshly to an offer of help.

In this case, we can have feelings of rejection. We will fear for our loved one's health, knowing that untreated depression can lead to dire consequences. Then, too, there can be consequences personally for us, if behaviors and moods due to depression intrude into our own lives.

Reacting with anger or withdrawing from the person in an attempt at self-preservation could be the only way we deal with our loved one's refusal to get treatment.

If our loved one refuses to consider treatment, we must give careful attention to boundaries and limitations. A person can't be forced to seek treatment. This decision is his or hers. What we can do is to offer support, love, and encouragement. We can make observations, provide information, and keep watch for a more serious downturn. Refusing treatment may seem bewildering, causing us pain as we watch so much suffering. But we have to draw the line between the depressed person and ourselves.

This is a time when we need to recall our PACT with our Higher Power. We need affirmation in the face of rejection of an offer to care and be present. We need the community of supportive friends and relatives to help us as we may be forced to watch a downward spiral—and we need prayer to help us stay in relationship with that Higher Power, who loves us through the dark times.

Meditation

"Love is the only game that is not called on account of darkness."

Thomas Carlyle

Everything we know of through our sense of sight relies upon degrees of light and darkness. We need light to function. With the coming of night, activity slows or even stops. School days end, businesses close, streets become empty. Most of us head to bed, giving up on the day that's passed to surrender to the comfort of sleep.

The darkness brought about by depression means a slowing down of activity, an emptiness of soul. When we care deeply for someone who is depressed, darkness threatens to break our relationship. Only love, consciously and deliberately kept alive and active, can overcome such darkness.

Recalling the love we have experienced from our Higher Power can be the one shaft of light keeping us from giving in to despair when we see a loved one slipping away from us due to depression. In gratitude to our Higher Power for the love and acceptance we've been given, we can find the patience and strength to continue to love when the darkness of depression descends.

Thank you for your unconditional love
when I am difficult to love. Give me the
ability to love others in the same way.

Armed with Information

When you begin to assist your loved one in finding effective treatment, the enormity of the task is often overwhelming. One way to increase your confidence is to arm yourself with as much information as possible. We need to know about different types of medications, different types of therapists, costs, and health care coverage. The more we know, the better assistance we're able to give.

If at all possible, research the illness before you get started making appointments. Whether you turn to a clergy person, a friend who's faced similar difficulties, or a trusted physician, you need to get as much guidance as you can from those who live in your community and are familiar with available resources. Locate the website for the particular health plan in question and study the benefits guide. Make use of customer service phone numbers for specific questions about types of treatment covered (or partially covered).

A little basic background information can help you as well. Though it may be tempting to jump onto a search engine and devour as much as you can find on the Internet, please remember that good information can be difficult to distinguish from bad information. Personal bias and commercial interests abound on many websites. Be discriminating as you research information about depression, and always temper information you receive even from the most accurate and reliable websites by any guidance you receive from a trusted physician, psychologist, psychiatrist, or therapist.

Reliable, accurate, and up-to-date information about depression and treatments can be found from these websites:

- www.mayoclinic.com

  The Mayo Clinic has long been recognized worldwide as a leader in medical research and treatment. Their website consistently wins awards for accuracy and trustworthy health information. Included on the website is a thorough discussion of different types of mental health providers, which can be helpful in selecting a therapist.

- www.nimh.nih.gov

  The National Institute of Mental Health is a leader in the area of research and treatment of mental illness.

- www.nami.org

  The National Alliance on Mental Illness provides information and support to those with mental illnesses and their families and friends. In addition, NAMI provides a helpline (1-800-950-NAMI) with trained volunteers who can provide information, referrals, and support.

- www.cdc.gov

  The Centers for Disease Control and Prevention is a federal agency that provides information to protect and promote public health and safety.

Antidepressant Medications

Antidepressants target various chemicals in the brain, such as serotonin and dopamine, and are believed to elevate mood. They can take several weeks to reach effective levels. Adjustments in dosage are often necessary, and sometimes more than one medication might be combined to achieve the best results. Side effects to watch for should be discussed with the prescribing doctor. These medications should never be stopped abruptly without consulting with the prescribing doctor. It's usually necessary to ramp down slowly to avoid serious side effects from withdrawal.

Antidepressants that are available include:

- **Selective serotonin reuptake inhibitors (SSRIs)**
  Some of the most heavily advertised medications are included in this category. SSRIs are often the first course of medication recommended.

- **Serotonin and norepinephrine reuptake inhibitors (SNRIs)**

- **Norepinephrine and dopamine reuptake inhibitors (NDRIs)**

- **Tricyclic antidepressants**
  Tricyclics have been available for a number of years, and are often suggested if SSRIs are found to be ineffective.

- **Monoamine oxidase inhibitors (MAOIs)**
  Because MAOIs require dietary restrictions and can have serious side effects, they are generally considered a last resort in depression treatment.

Types of Mental Health Professionals

Designations for a variety of mental health professionals, as well as the requirements for licensing, vary from state to state. Those described here are the most common terms. Other options exist, also varying from state to state.

Psychologist—Psychologists hold advanced degrees and provide therapy for a wide range of mental disorders. Their background includes training in diagnosis, assessment, many types of psychotherapy, and much more.

Licensed Clinical Social Worker (LCSW)—LCSWs are social workers with training in psychotherapy and many hours of clinical practice. They're able to help patients deal with a variety of mental health and daily living issues, often using a practical approach to improving the ability to function healthily.

Psychiatrist—Psychiatrists are medical doctors with a specialized background in mental disorders, and are able to prescribe antidepressant medications. General practitioners can also prescribe antidepressants, but do not have the same specialized field of study.

Psychopharmacologist—A psychopharmacologist is a medical doctor who is a psychiatrist but has extensively studied the medications used in dealing with depression. A psychopharmacologist is able to combine medications for the most effective treatment.

Some Therapy Options

There are many types of therapy employed by various mental health professionals. These are some of the most common.

Interpersonal

Interpersonal therapy, according to the National Association of Mental Illness, is a successful therapy approach for treating depression. It's focus is on improving difficult personal relationships and on adapting to changes in life that may have been associated with a person's depression.

Psychodynamic

Psychodynamic therapy is also commonly used in depression treatment. This type of therapy focuses on the underlying psychological basis for the suffering of the depressed person. According to the American Psychological

Association, self-reflection and self-examination are the distinguishing features of this form of therapy, which uses the relationship between therapist and patient as a window into problematic relationship patterns in the patient's life.

Cognitive Behavioral

Cognitive behavioral therapy, according to the National Association of Mental Illness, "helps to change the negative thinking and unsatisfying behavior associated with depression, while teaching people how to unlearn the behavioral patterns that contribute to their illness."

Other Treatments for Depression

Though a combination of medication and therapy is the most commonly recommended treatment, other options do exist.

In cases of severe depression over time with no relief found through traditional approaches, a medical procedure called Electroconvulsive Therapy (ECT) can be effective. ECT applies electric current to the brain, sometimes producing immediate relief of depression symptoms. Though at one time ECT was considered dangerous and barbaric, advances in the procedure have made it a good alternative when other treatments don't produce results.

St. John's wort has long been used as a treatment for depression. According to the Mayo Clinic, this herb has been proven to be more effective in fighting mild depression than a placebo, and possibly as effective as tricyclic antidepressants. However, it can create negative interactions with prescription medications (including SSRIs), other herbs, and supplements, and can elevate blood pressure. Therefore, anyone considering trying St. John's wort is advised to first consult a physician.

Then, too, some depressed individuals seek relief of symptoms through prayer, and there are some studies that support the health benefits of doing so. Other depressed persons may choose not to intervene medically on their own behalf in the belief that their Higher Power will heal them. Seeking the best treatment for depression is a difficult journey, with a unique path to improvement for each person. But recovery is possible.

Frustrations During the Treatment Process

As much as we may care for someone who is dealing with depression, the fact remains that the illness makes people hard to deal with. The list of symptoms itself creates a picture of a person whose behavior is likely to make us uncomfortable at the very least. When we've chosen to step in and be a partner in the treatment process, another level of frustration can be added.

Here we are, trying to help a person feel better, and it seems he or she doesn't want to feel better. He or she may be:

- too fatigued to follow up with doctor appointments,

- too forgetful to take medications on schedule,

- too confused to report whether he or she is experiencing improvement or any negative side effects,

- too irritable to express thanks for the time, effort, and love you're offering, or,

- all of the above.

We just have to develop a thick skin, and keep telling ourselves that this person we're seeing is not the person we've known and loved. Sometimes another decision must be made in our own minds—do we continue to keep following up on treatment steps, or do we back off and see what happens? It's a difficult, frustrating process, and we have to allow ourselves forgiveness and space when we feel things aren't going well.

Meditation

*"Our fatigue is often caused not by work, but
by worry, frustration, and resentment."*

Dale Carnegie*

Picture a hamster running on a wheel. It stretches its tiny legs out as far as it can, moving faster and faster, as if it could get somewhere if only it worked hard enough. Living long-term with a depressed person can feel like an endless run on a hamster wheel. We move faster and faster, trying to get somewhere, trying to make something change, but the faster we run, the more we stay in the same place. Life with a depressed partner creates frustrations that make us want to drop in exhaustion. Real and painful circumstances create the feeling that we are trapped inside a cage.

In the face of such exhausting frustration, rest is a necessity. The best gift we can give ourselves is to step off the wheel for a time. This rest time can take whatever form is best for us, from a good book to music to coffee with a friend—whatever distracts us enough to keep our minds off those frustrations for a time. As we rest, refresh, and restore, we are better able to engage in time with our Higher Power, sharing our frustrations, listening for peace and comfort. Rest, prayer, and an intentional change of focus can slow down the speed of the wheel, for our own health and well-being.

*Higher Power, help me find a way and a
time to step off the endless cycle of frustration
and share with You a time of rest.*

---

* Used by permission of Dale Carnegie Institute.

Try This

When in the coming week can you find a time of rest so you can change focus? Block out a time (even if it's only ten minutes) in which you can step off your wheel of frustration and do something for yourself.

Keeping Track of Progress

People in active depression are generally incapable of managing their own course of treatment. Perhaps they're unable to recall what medication and what dosage they're currently taking, let alone what medications they've tried in the past. They forget helpful strategies suggested by a therapist, and therefore never even get around to trying them. They might not recognize when their moods begin to lift, or when symptoms begin to abate.

Because it can be so very difficult for a depressed person to keep up with his or her own treatment, we can do a great service by keeping track for them. If we have the time and energy to keep a log of medications, dosages, appointments, behavioral strategies, and observed behavior and moods, this assistance can prove to be invaluable in the recovery process.

Try This

Copy the following pages for use in keeping track of your loved one's progress. Because treatment is such a trial-and-error process, you're likely to need a number of copies over a period of time.

Date:

Medication Notes

Current medication(s):

Dosage:

Name of prescribing doctor:

Prescribing doctor contact information:

Last appointment with prescribing doctor:

Next scheduled appointment with prescribing doctor:

Any side effects noted:

Any mood or symptom changes noted:

Questions, comments, or topics to bring up at next appointment: ....

....

....

Therapy Session Notes

Therapist's name: ....

Therapist contact information: ....

Last appointment with therapist: ....

Next scheduled appointment with therapist: ....

Any coping strategies suggested by therapist: ....

....

How often has _____ tried this coping strategy? ....

Has any success been noted with this strategy? ....

....

Any mood or symptom changes noted: ....

....

Questions, comments, or topics to bring up at next therapy appointment: ......

....

Finding our way through the darkness of depression is a long, difficult process. It's a true act of love to willingly embark on this journey with a depressed person. Be sure to give yourself the grace to make mistakes, to become frustrated, to acknowledge your own limitations. Give yourself credit for doing the best you can in a very painful situation, and keep yourself in relationship with your Higher Power, who knows better than we ever can what it means to be near and present in all times, good and bad, light and dark.

CHAPTER THREE NOTES

1. U.S. Centers for Disease Control and Prevention. 2005. *CDC: Antidepressants Most Prescribed Drugs in U.S.* [Online]. Available from http://edition.cnn.com/2007/HEALTH/07/09antidepressants/index.html (accessed 10 July 2010).

2. IMS Health Reports. 2008. *U.S. Prescription Sales Grew 3.8 Percent in 2007, to $286.5 Billion* [Online]. Available from http://www.imshealth.com/portal/site/imshealth/menuitem.a46c6d4df3d b4b3d88f611019418c22a/?vgnextoid=280c1d3be7a29110VgnVCM10000071812ca2RCRD&vg nextchannel=41a67900b55a5110VgnVCM10000071812ca2RCRD&vgnextfmt=default (accessed 11 May 2011).

3. Department of Health and Human Services Substance Abuse and Mental Health Services Administration (SAMHSA) Office of Applied Studies (OAS). 2008. *Results from the 2007 National Survey on Drug Use and Health: National Findings* [Online]. Available from http://oas.samhsa.gov/NSDUH/2k7nsduh/2k7results.cfm#Ch8 (accessed 29 July 2010).

CHAPTER FOUR

Relationships and Changing the Dance Steps

"If instead of a gem, or even a flower, we should cast the gift of a loving thought into the heart of a friend, that would be giving as the angels give."

George MacDonald

In Steven Cleaver's novel *Saving Erasmus*, a newly ordained minister, Andrew Benoit, has to come to terms with the changing relationships in his life before he can begin to consider saving an entire town. He struggles with all the challenges and changes that abound in his life, wrestling most with his fear of abandonment. When he reaches the point where he no longer fears, but embraces, the changes in his relationships, he is able to face himself and save the people of Erasmus.

It is no different when one deals with depression. We who live day in and day out with those struggling with this illness must learn to face that which we fear the most—the loss of our loved one to the black hole of despair and the loss of the person we came to love.

Meditation

*"Just as driving on the correct side of the
road gives us the freedom to go anywhere,
so accepting the natural law of constant
change is our route to freedom."*

Adapted from teachings of the Buddha

"We've always done it that way."

"It won't be the same."

"I don't like change."

We've all heard or said these same words time and time
again. Being creatures of habit, we like the comfort of
changelessness. We like knowing where things are. We
pride ourselves on knowing what to expect from family
and friends. When those expectations are not met, it often
throws us into turmoil.

"Why isn't Johnny laughing like he used to?"

"Why isn't Mom keeping the place clean? She's always been
such a neat freak."

"What happened to Mike after the baby came? He was
looking forward to being a good father, and now he's
acting like the child doesn't mean anything to him."

When the people in our lives change, it can make us
think that something is wrong, because our relationship is
different and we want it to go back to "normal." But there
is no "normal." Life is ever-changing, and our relationships

are ever-changing, too. How we relate to one another, what we see in one another changes each and every day. The sometimes-dramatic changes created by depression make us feel threatened. We want our old relationship back. Perhaps, when we recognize that everything changes, we may be able to look at the changes depression brings as a new way to understand our friends, families, and partners better. We might not like the changes, we might not understand the changes, but when we stick to the right side of the road, we are able to be free to explore this new side of our loved ones without fear or resentment. We might be better able to help them and ourselves with this change, however surprising or unwelcome it may be.

Lord, help me to be ever-open to change
and to see the new in everyone.

Kaleidoscope of Relationships

No one is ever in just one relationship; we live in relationships with many people, and those relationships have an impact on one another. At any one time we can be parent, spouse, sibling, daughter, partner, teacher, coworker, friend, neighbor, cousin, roommate. The list is as long as the number of people we know. Our lives are lived through relationship—from our interaction with the checkout person at the grocery store to conversation with a husband when he comes home from work.

We approach our many relationships differently, and each relationship hinges on others. If we exchange harsh words with the clerk at the store, we might take that ugliness home with us. We argue with our spouse, who then is grumpy with the kids, who in turn start to bicker with one another. What started out as a minor irritation can send a day, and several relationships, into a tailspin.

Our relationships change day in and day out. We drift away from people due to circumstances, misunderstandings, or serious differences of opinion. We draw closer to others through shared experiences, through common interests, or simply due to the amount of time spent together. If we can't recognize and adapt to these changes, many problems can result—smaller problems in more casual relationships, and large problems in relationships that are important to us. When changes are the result of the presence of depression, enormous pressures affect multiple aspects of our lives. It is only by dealing with changes, no how matter how difficult they may be, that we are able to maintain the essence of our valued relationships.

"Mighty God, Father of all,
Compassionate God, Mother of all,
bless every person I have met,
every face I have seen,
every voice I have heard,
especially those most dear;
bless every city, town and street I have known,
bless every sight I have seen,
every sound I have heard,
every object I have touched.
in some mysterious way these
have all fashioned my life;
all that I am,
I have received.
Great God, bless the world."

"God Bless the World" John J. Morris, S.J.[*]

The Marriage Relationship

Jane and Tom had been married for twenty-five years. During that time they were happy raising two children, with professional lives that were fulfilling for each of them. Tom had always suffered from dysthymia, low-grade depression present from childhood, and both of them were used to periods of time when Tom functioned less well than in others. During these bouts, he slept for longer periods of time and preferred to spend time with friends rather than family. These episodes, however, would be fairly short, and through talking with Jane, Tom was able to move beyond them and back to their normal, comfortable routine.

The problems started when Tom took to sleeping the day away. He stayed in bed until noon or later, got up to eat lunch, worked at his desk for half an hour or less, and then returned to bed, waking only to say "hi" to the kids after school and to take care of bathroom needs. When Jane approached him to talk about these changes, he became sullen and told her to mind her own business, accusing her of lacking patience. This was so different from their usual dance that Jane didn't know quite how to react. As days went by and nothing changed, she felt more and more distant from Tom. She discussed the situation with a friend. Why doesn't he want to talk with me about it? Why, suddenly, has his sleeping pattern changed? Why doesn't he show any interest in me or the kids? It was only when her friend asked her if she had asked herself the question, "What is he trying to tell me?" that Jane saw the situation in a new light.

Jane recognized, through talking with her doctor and with trusted friends, that Tom was experiencing more serious depression than ever before. With their kids leaving for college and a job he enjoyed less and less all the time, he no longer felt that life was full of promise. The low-grade depression he had felt all of his life was now moving into a major depression and had to be dealt with in a completely different way.

In a marriage relationship, two people begin a life together with promises to each other and expectations of each other. Generally two married people hope to settle into a pattern of relating to each other that is comfortable and allows them to grow and mature through life together. A mutual dependence grows out of years of marriage, over issues as complicated as emotional support or as mundane as household tasks. The presence of depression can throw mutual dependence and patterns of behavior into a tailspin. The nondepressed spouse can end up feeling bereft due to the loss of comfort and companionship.

Older-Parent-and-Adult-Child Caregiver Relationship

When Julie began to take care of her mother following a slight stroke, she was not prepared for what took place. Julie's mom Esther had been an active woman. She regularly went out with friends to lunch or coffee, played bridge, belonged to a book club, and enjoyed time with her grandchildren. All of that seemed to change overnight. Esther no longer wanted to see her grandchildren, let alone play with them. When Esther did interact with them, Julie had to spend a great deal of time soothing the hurt feelings of the grandchildren, who were stung by the harsh words of their grandmother. Esther was still physically able to read, but would not finish a book, tossing one after another aside and making sweeping judgments about their contents. When Julie tried to interest her mother in a book she had read and enjoyed, the older woman sneered that Julie wasn't well-read enough to make an insightful recommendation. It was a heartbreaking time.

Julie didn't like the changes she saw in her mother, but she was smart enough to know these changes didn't have to be permanent. After talking with a psychopharmacologist, she was able to arrange for an examination that resulted in her mother being prescribed antidepressant medication, and soon Esther was back to her old self. Actually, she experienced a new-and-improved self because she had realized her behavior was unpleasant, but had felt unable to do anything about it.

As the general population ages, the medical community recognizes that depressed people who are elderly are chronically undertreated. Faced with failing bodies, the loss of friends, the distance of family members, and perhaps entry into an assisted-living or nursing home, many elderly people find themselves in a situation that sets the stage for depression. No longer able to take care of themselves or interact with people who are genuinely interested in them, they live among people who are paid to fill their basic needs but who have no real interest in them as persons, as individuals.

This is a time of life when people are going through changes—metabolic shifts, chemical rebalancing, and dropping of serotonin levels, all of which can affect mood and influence the development of depression. Add to that physical maladies or accidents and the problem is compounded.

Same-Sex Partnerships

Jenny and Andrea had been in a relationship for more than four years. They'd met in a neighborhood tavern during the weekly trivia night. They hit it off over a number of common interests, and soon were living together and very happy. About a year into their union, however, Andrea began to act "funny." Whereas before she would eagerly introduce Jenny to friends and coworkers, she now would go out of her way to avoid having Jenny meet anyone from her social circles. When circumstances compelled her to introduce Jenny, she always said she was "a friend" and never used the term "partner."

Andrea then began to go out of her way to meet men, even hooking up with a guy after a night of particularly heavy drinking. She came home and told Jenny that it was the best sex she had ever had. When Andrea's mother died a few weeks later, Andrea was convinced she was being punished for her relationship with Jenny. Jenny didn't know what to do. She loved Andrea but the craziness of the past few months was getting to her and she began to question how strong her love for Andrea was.

Jenny finally talked Andrea into going to one counseling session together. That's all Andrea would agree to. During the session, Andrea's fears of rejection by loved ones and her self-hatred based on years of hiding her authentic nature from the world tumbled out. Healing and understanding were able to begin. Andrea wasn't sure she would go back to therapy, but having agreed to go once was a positive step.

The vast majority of gay men and lesbian women, according to mental health surveys, are out to family and close friends—97.6 and 86.3 percent, respectively. This openness within a close community can be extremely helpful in dealing with the different challenges that depression poses for gay couples. Unfortunately, gay and lesbian people often must cope with homophobia, institutional and otherwise, and with bullying that may have occurred in childhood (and beyond), legal inequities, lack of acceptance and understanding, and a societal stigma that, while lessening, has not completely disappeared.

Roommates

Aden and Grant were roommates at an elite school in the Northeast. They hadn't known each other until moving-in day of their freshman year. They hit it off immediately, negotiating the best arrangement for their dorm room. Classes began, and each one started to make his own friends, knowing that they had each other to fall back on. They spent some evenings gaming together and occasionally went out for pizza. It wasn't an intimate relationship, but they cared about each other as friends.

Around Halloween, Aden started to notice that Grant's bed hadn't been slept in several mornings a week, or he would come in at three or four in the morning, smelling of alcohol, and collapse on the bed. Aden wondered when Grant was getting his work done and when was he eating. As the days progressed, it became evident that Grant was not doing his schoolwork. There had been several calls from the dean of his school and several unanswered calls from his parents. One morning, Aden waited until Grant got up from yet another binge and asked him how he was doing. Grant immediately turned on Aden, fists raised. "Keep the hell out of my business," he snarled, and stomped off. Aden didn't know what to do. Something was wrong, but should he get involved? He talked with his counselor, changed rooms, and from then on saw Grant only in passing. Aden didn't feel good about this end to their relationship, but it was the only solution he could see.

Rooming together can be inherently difficult. Clear lines of involvement or lack of involvement may never be fully delineated, even in relationships that do not carry the cloud of depression. With depression in the picture, it becomes a game of trying to figure out when something should be said and when it shouldn't. It becomes a challenge trying to determine whether the depressed person is in danger or whether to break confidence and look for help. In addition, it's very difficult for an emotionally healthy roommate to live in a small room with a depressed person who is unpredictable in mood and behavior.

Intimate Partners

Craig and Carol had dated for several months when they decided to take their relationship a step further. Neither felt ready for marriage, but they cared enough for each other that they wanted a more serious commitment. They found an apartment to share and enjoyed living together for nearly a year. Right after their first anniversary of moving in together, though, Craig started making a habit of having a few drinks every evening. Before long he progressed to drinking himself to sleep three or four nights a week, passing out in his clothes on the couch. Carol was at a loss. Any attempts to suggest the existence of a drinking problem led to argument. She didn't know Craig's parents well enough to feel comfortable calling them. Though she cared for Craig and cherished the time they'd had together, soon she was thinking seriously of moving out and getting herself out of a relationship she hadn't bargained for.

Add romantic love into the mix when two people live together, and a relationship becomes ever more complicated. The degree of involvement is a bit more clear-cut than for platonic roommates, but the commitment may not be solid enough for one person to step in to help the other if depression makes the situation perilous or life-threatening. Mentioning uncharacteristic behavior or bringing up serious concerns can lead to arguments that either break the relationship or place the advocate in a very difficult situation.

Children, Parents, and Friends

Fia was a bright, happy girl of five. She enjoyed running and jumping and playing with her dolls. She loved picking flowers. With a bright, engaging smile and a bubbling laugh, she was able to engage even the grumpiest of adults in conversation. Sometimes at night Fia became sad when she overheard her mother and father arguing—but in the morning, when she would find them at the breakfast table with smiles for her, that made everything better.

One morning, she went downstairs for breakfast and found her mother and father arguing. They didn't notice her, and when she tried to interrupt them her father angrily pushed her aside. Fia backed into a corner and watched in horror as her father hit her mother again and again. He didn't stop until her mother fell to the floor—and he didn't turn to Fia to reassure her everything would be all right, as he had before.

At that moment Fia began the journey into darkness. She didn't understand what had happened. She only knew it made her afraid. Even when her mother felt better and tried to reassure her, Fia only felt fear. Soon she was no longer smiling or laughing. She wouldn't pick flowers, and often she would come home, go up to her room, take one of her dolls, and very slowly and systematically break it into pieces. It took an observant teacher to get help for Fia. When her mother and father joined her in family therapy, she was finally able to begin to heal.

There are many theories about why the statistics on children and depression are climbing. Some blame technology, others the stress of an overscheduled childhood. Still others say it is the breakdown of our society. Sometimes, just as in adults, a chemical imbalance is present that creates depression. But there has been comparatively little research on depression in young children. There are common threads that do run through the histories of children with depression. They include a life lived with too many stressors. Another thread is instability in the family. Children pick up on tension and stress and often react with depression when their safe home is invaded by problems. For older children and adolescents, drugs and alcohol may play a part in depression, although it's a case of the proverbial chicken and egg—which comes first, substance abuse or depression?

Depression is not only an adult problem. Children might not react with symptoms in the same way that adults do. They might act out of character, perhaps becoming irritable or extremely placating. Grades may drop; kids may isolate themselves or spend more and more time unaccounted for. Any questionable symptoms in children should be considered carefully in case they indicate clinical depression.

Recognizing and Monitoring Changing Relationships

Lists of depression symptoms are commonly found in magazine articles and advertisements, on websites, on talk shows—and in books like this one. Such checklists can be helpful in recognizing that a problem is present. What can truly shock us, though, and what are usually not alluded to in the ads or on the websites or talk shows, are the unusual behaviors triggered by depression. Even when we're aware of what depression can do to a person, we can be caught totally unaware when our loved one does something that seems bizarre. Also surprising to people with a depressed loved one are the personality changes that can manifest themselves. Books and lists can't fully describe what we actually experience when someone we care for is depressed.

Unusual and shocking behaviors triggered by depression must, we realize, stem from great pain in our loved one. We hurt to see them in this pain, and the pain affects us as well, through altered and unusual behaviors. Daily life can be disrupted by the confusion and crisis brought on by a loved one's depression. Not only do we have to witness their pain and suffering, but we suffer direct consequences ourselves.

No two relationships experience depression in the same way. Growing up, we were always told that no two snowflakes were the same. That adage goes for the way depression works in a relationship. Nothing is guaranteed except the darkness of the disease. Still, when people who love the depressed person are able to navigate the turmoil, truth and goodness can result from the experience. However, we must expect change and we must monitor the change and how it affects us.

Commonly Observed Behaviors, Attitudes, or Other Manifestations of Depression That May Affect Loved One(s)

Lethargy

Your spouse, who had formerly been an equal partner in housework, completely stops participating in chores. When you come home late from work, your husband, who has been home all day, has left you a kitchen full of dirty dishes, a bedroom piled with dirty clothes, overflowing trash cans, no groceries on the shelves, and a litter box that hasn't been changed in days. On one level you understand—lack of energy is a common symptom of depression. But the reality of living with someone who appears to be a lazy slob not only makes you angry, it keeps you up late each night trying to clean up the detritus of daily life.

Difficulty making decisions

You're running late for a movie, but you're both starving. First it takes a fifteen-minute discussion to decide where to stop for fast food—annoying enough in itself. Then, when you get to the counter to place an order, your friend keeps you and everyone else in line waiting for a full ten minutes more, trying to decide what to put on her hamburger and which soft drink to get. Not only are you made hopelessly late for the show, you're embarrassed by her behavior and by the sounds of impatience you hear in the customers in line behind you.

Excessive sleeping/change in sleeping habits

Mom, who moved in with you when her depression took over, has become nocturnal. She's up through most of the night, disrupting your sleep because lights and television are on in the living room until all hours. She sleeps most of the day, and is just getting up when you come home after work. The poor quality of sleep you're experiencing shows itself in your shortened temper, and seriously increases your embarrassment factor when you bring a coworker home for supper one evening, to be greeted by your bleary-eyed mother in pajamas and bathrobe on the couch in front of the television.

Changes in sexual expression

Various changes can occur in the sexual expression of an intimate relationship. Sex, as a satisfying and meaningful part of a relationship, can disappear completely or become very intermittent. Medication taken for the depression might complicate this issue. Perhaps you can't remember being touched in weeks. You're left feeling hurt, lonely, and frustrated. You question whether you're no longer attractive, if he or she is having an affair, or if you are no longer loved. You might discover that your loved one has turned to pornography, has indeed begun an affair, or has resorted to long calls to a sex hotline. On the other hand, you may suddenly find your depressed loved one cannot get enough intimate time with you. Most of these choices are the depressed person's manifestation of physical and emotional needs and exhaustion. Still, when any of this happens, it can hurt deeply.

Unexplained physical problems

Your twenty-six-year-old son has moved back home after losing his job due to a bout of depression. Not only are you needed to keep him on track with depression medications and therapy sessions, but he's constantly ill, achy, or complaining of physical issues that you're afraid not to follow up on. He can't manage to get to the doctor's office on his own, and over time you've become his schedule manager, chauffeur, and nurse—all of which eats up your free time and your energy.

To Sum Up

If someone you love is depressed, then chances are one or more of these behavioral changes sounds at least slightly familiar to you. The degree to which these types of changes are affecting you personally, as a loved one and caregiver, depends on the closeness of your relationship, the depth of the depression, and other factors. What is a constant, however, for those of us who are in relationship with a depressed person is that our own lives, too, are affected deeply by the illness.

Reflections

- *What specific issues and behavioral changes related to my loved one's depression are affecting me the most?*

- *In what ways am I being affected?*

Hurdling Communication Barriers

One of the earliest casualties in a relationship affected by depression is the ability to communicate. Many of the symptoms of depression—confusion, memory loss, irritability—create barriers to the give-and-take, the listening and sharing required in effective communication. There's truth in the saying "Communication is a two-way street." When one of the people involved is depressed, that street easily becomes one-way, leading to a dead end.

Jan and Eric, having lived together for three years, had been dealing with Jan's depression for several months. Though Jan was struggling, they decided to take a summer trip to visit Eric's family, a cross-country trip requiring a lot of planning and discussion. Days before their departure date, Jan's behavior made Eric question whether they would be able to manage the trip. Any time he wanted to discuss it with Jan, he had to try over and over again even to get her attention. From one day to the next she forgot details of the trip: how far they planned to drive the first day, which car they'd decided to take, what the plans were when they arrived. Trying to help her feel involved and raise her interest level, he suggested she plan a scenic route for part of the trip—something she had always enjoyed in the past. This discussion itself was tricky, as Jan snapped at Eric for repeating himself when it appeared she didn't understand him. To make matters worse, Eric was hurt to find on checking back with Jan the next day that not only had she forgotten to look at the map, she didn't even recall that she was supposed to plan a route. It seemed as if Jan didn't care about their vacation at all. The fun and anticipation of the trip were spoiled in Eric's mind.

Life with a depressed person is full of such miscommunications and hurt feelings. Attempts at conversation are cut off when our loved one lacks energy and focus. Things we feel are important are forgotten due to struggles with memory. The grouchiness that accompanies the illness feels like a slap in the face. Before long, we give up even trying to communicate.

There are a few things we can do to head off some of these difficult issues. A good place to start is to continually and intentionally remind yourself that the way your loved one reacts when you're talking is not a personal attack, though it may come off that way. When frustrated or hurt in attempts at conversation, separate yourself from the situation as soon as possible—

count to ten, find an excuse to end the discussion for a time, change the subject, whatever it takes. While taking a break, reassess the necessity of the conversation; sometimes avoiding and "working around" is a reasonable option. Consider alternate ways or times to approach the subject, as well. Many depressed people have predictable patterns to their day, times when they're more coherent and perhaps more energetic. Planning important conversations around this time can help.

When you need your loved one to remember something you've discussed, create a system of reminders for him or her. Ask what would be most helpful—notes, emails, phone messages, texts, a combination of these? Work to ensure that this system doesn't seem like nagging; rather, it's a way for the two of you to maintain a good relationship.

Communication may continue to be a one-way street as long as depression is present. But with some deliberate effort on your part, you can keep the traffic on that street moving at a pace you can live with.

Dealing with Depression's Effects

Living with and supporting someone through depression is not easy. It's difficult to keep learning new dance steps to an old song. It's difficult to maintain a relationship, particularly if only one person is working at it because the other doesn't have the strength. During times like this we need to know that love is not an emotion; rather, love is a decision, a choice we freely make day after day, and sometimes hour after hour or minute to minute. We can choose to love even when a person seems rather unloveable. We choose to work with our loved one as he or she struggles through depression. Choosing to love in the face of depression is not easy. Often it is only through enlisting the help of our Higher Power, who we know loves us through even the worst times, that we find the strength to love someone else through the worst.

Pause to remember what makes your relationship with the depressed person so special to you. Recall times when you felt happy about each other. In short, take a pause from all the "stuff" that is coming at you, and remember—remember your loved one in better days, remember the presence of your Higher Power, remember that this too will pass.

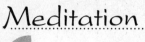Meditation

"I like not only to be loved, but
also to be told I am loved."

George Eliot

Sometimes couples judge the healthiness of their relationship by the frequency of sex. When sex is good, many of us tend to think that the relationship is on solid ground. However, when depression becomes a third party, using the bedroom as a gauge of love can cause a number of problems.

Sexual acts can be beautiful demonstrations of the love that already exists in a relationship. Of course, there are also many other ways to express love—thoughtful actions, a listening ear, a caress in times of trouble. Unfortunately, depression tends to rob a relationship of these forms of loving attention. When that happens, we may begin to think of sex as the only way love can be expressed. Instead, we need to look at the whole of the relationship and see the expressions of love throughout our lives together. We need to listen to those moments that tell us that we are appreciated and if it weren't for us, the road of depression would be much more difficult. We can recognize the small, loving gestures our partner offers when he or she is feeling good on a particular day. Though these acts may be small or infrequent, our hearts need to stay open to the evidence of the love that still exists in the relationship.

Open my eyes to the acts of love that permeate my life.

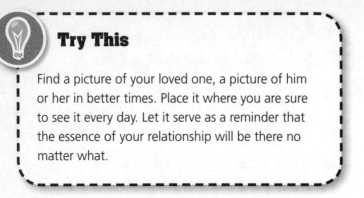

Try This

Find a picture of your loved one, a picture of him or her in better times. Place it where you are sure to see it every day. Let it serve as a reminder that the essence of your relationship will be there no matter what.

Stepping away from the pain and hurt of changed relationships can help to prepare us for the issues that tend to affect us, and can help us maintain a healthy sense of balance. Though it can be difficult to stand back and recognize where problems are arising and what we can do to head them off, it's worth the effort. Consider using a formal system for assessing your situation. Think about how changes are affecting the depressed individual, and how they are affecting those around him or her. Are changed behaviors destructive, or are they potentially enriching? Might the behaviors be a temporary response to a new medication or an event, or do they seem to have become part of the fabric of the individual's being? Such questions help to determine whether changes that are seen and experienced need immediate response or they can be observed and responded to as a changing part of the individual's personality.

Try This

For your own well-being, monitor the ways your loved one's depression affects you. Photocopying the following page and filling it out periodically can help you keep track of your own state.

How _____'s
Depression Affects Me

Date: _____

Negative behaviors created by depression that
occurred today: _____
_____
_____
_____

How I felt:_____
_____
_____
_____

What I did in response: _____
_____
_____
_____

Has this happened before?_____
_____
_____
_____

Possible action to take if this happens again:_____
_____
_____
_____

Starting Over Again ... and Again

When we've invested time, emotion, and energy in a relationship, radical changes due to a partner's depression may force us to reevaluate our commitment. In some cases, perhaps when two people live together but are not married, or when we can no longer keep up with an emotional roller coaster created by a friend's depression, the best solution may be to break off the relationship and move on.

But in a relationship with legal, moral, or "blood" ties, such as that of parent/child, life partners, or spouses, there may be added determination to keep the relationship alive. In this case, it can help to adopt the action of continually looking at your loved one in a new and different light, realizing that they might be at different emotional places at any given point in time. Turn the kaleidoscope and look at your situation through new eyes. Yes, the relationship is different, and it might remain different for a while. It also might never go back to being the way it was. If indeed this was a relationship that was deeply mutually satisfying, then the relationship in its new form will be worth preserving. When we choose to love, we choose it with all of its dimensions—the pain, the good times, the confusion—and we are ever-grateful for the changes that free us to grow into a deeper relationship.

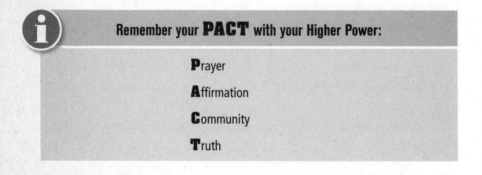

Remember your **PACT** with your Higher Power:

Prayer

Affirmation

Community

Truth

When the person with whom we choose to be in relationship has depression, we're choosing the possibility of committing ourselves to someone who may appear to be a different person from day to day. This fluid state of affairs requires us to be willing to start over each time changes become apparent. It requires us to look for positives in someone who seems negative most of the time. It probably requires, too, the help of a Higher Power—we're unlikely to have the strength within ourselves to take on this challenge without help and guidance. The "P" of PACT can be of great comfort when we make the choice to stay in the relationship. From prayer we can find strength and energy to get through whatever depression might do to our loved one from one day to the next.

Reflections

- *How can I recommit to my loved one?*

- *What am I able to do to bring stability into the relationship?*

- *Who can help me during this struggle?*

- *What is good about my relationship right now?*

- *What new thing have I learned about my loved one?*

A Ceremony of Recommitment

Gather around you those individuals you love and who have supported you and your loved one during this difficult time. Ask them all to join hands around you and your loved one, who remain in the middle of the circle as one of you reads or recites:

"We come today to recognize the changes that have taken place in our relationship.

These changes have not affected the love we have for each other. These changes have not taken away the surprise and wonder we have for each other. Instead, these changes have opened for us wondrous new opportunities to discover what each of us is and can be. These changes have deepened the love we have for each other and have called us to recommit to each other as we continue this journey of life."

Together the two in the circle say:

> "I want to be your friend
> Forever and ever without break or decay.
> When the hills are all flat
> And the rivers are all dry,
> When it lightens and thunders in winter,
> When it rains and snows in summer,
> When Heaven and Earth mingle—
> Not till then will I part from you."
> ———
> First-Century Chinese Oath of Friendship

The two in the circle hug while those in the larger circle step inward toward the center, in essence making a large hug. One of the two in the circle says:

> "I've read all the books, but
> Only one remains sacred:
> This volume of wonders, open
> Always before my eyes."
> ———
> Kathleen Raine[*]

"I recommit to you now, and with the help of my Higher Power, I always will. I love you."

---

[*] Used with permission by the estate of Kathleen Raine, Ipswich, Great Britain.

CHAPTER FIVE

Daily Life in the Dark

"The tragedy of life is not so much what men suffer, but rather what they miss."

Thomas Carlyle

The alarm clock rings, signaling the start of another day. When you live with someone who is suffering from depression, this can also be the signal of the start of a long struggle that lasts until you crawl back into bed for the night. When someone is depressed, daily life becomes a monumental struggle to deal with—regarding sleep, direction, finances, and ordinary day-to-day tasks. What would be simple decisions for a person without depression become life-changing choices for the person with depression. For those around him or her, it can mean exasperation, anger, and a feeling of being pulled down into the mire of darkness.

Time to Get Up

Getting out of bed in the morning is perhaps one of the most difficult things that some people with depression can do. It is far easier to ignore the dark cloud while one is sleeping rather than to have it ever-present during waking hours. Consequently, the day can start with a great deal of tension.

When the alarm went off in Joshua's room, he would simply turn over and pull the pillow over his head. He had nothing to do. He had nowhere to go. Why did he have to get up? His wife had died three months earlier. Joshua was okay through the funeral and the days immediately after, but as the weeks went on, he found that he missed the sense of purpose he'd found in caring for her. Now, at the age of seventy, he had nothing to do, no place to go.

His daughter, Janice, came to live with him when the doctor expressed concern about Joshua's ability to care for himself. She saw to his meals but got upset when he declined to eat. She thought he should go out for a walk each day, and when he balked at that, she balked right back. When he did go out, he found himself buying items he neither liked nor needed, but for a time he felt better because of his purchases. Janice was at wit's end, not knowing what to do or where to go. After a while she simply let him sleep until he was ready to get up—which sometimes was three in the afternoon—because the quiet was much better than the arguing.

Sleep needs vary—but approximately seven hours of sleep are what most adults need to function effectively, and for many eight to ten might be needed. However, when someone sleeps the day away, this is generally a red flag that something is wrong. Sleep disturbances—including both under- and oversleeping—are common symptoms of depression, and repeatedly sleeping the day away certainly indicates a serious problem. Sleep problems can exist, or surface, even after treatment has begun.

What is the nondepressed caregiver to do? A good place to start is to make sure medication is being taken as prescribed. People still in the grips of depression are often unable to recall when or whether they've taken their meds. Overmedication can send the patient's energy level into the pits, leading to excessive sleep. Undermedication can mean the symptoms of depression don't fully disappear, allowing abnormal sleep patterns to continue.

A daily pill organizer, carefully monitored by someone other than the depressed person, can be very helpful in this situation. If, in fact, medication has been taken correctly and on schedule, the next step is to visit the prescribing doctor as soon as possible. An adjustment—sometimes repeated adjustments—may be needed in order to reach the most effective level for the patient. Then, daily monitoring of the pill box and repeated check-ins must continue.

Encouraging an oversleeper to take small steps toward getting up can make a big difference as well. One of the things Lisa tried with her sister was to get her sister up when the alarm went off, helping her to get dressed and ready for the day. "She might not go anywhere or do anything except sit on the couch and stare or read, but she was up and that was a very small 'big' step. She was to some extent participating in the day."

Another way to handle oversleeping is found in Mark's story. When Mark's partner consistently stayed in bed long into the day, his frustration at this disruption of their lives began to turn to anger. At first, Mark found himself berating Brinda for being lazy, for being no help around the house when she was stuck in bed, for leaving the daily chores to him. One day, after finally rising at noon, Brinda was clearheaded enough to tell Mark that his angry words made it even harder for her to face the day. Saddened by the extra pain he'd caused her, Mark learned to bite back his anger and instead used gentle, encouraging words when it was time for Brinda to get up. Her waking schedule didn't instantly return to normal, but soon she was beginning to get out of bed and become alert earlier and earlier each day.

Meditation

"But I and those who loved me wondered why
such great persecution came upon me and
why God did not bring me comfort."

Hildegard of Bingen

Wondering "why" can sometimes be a full-time occupation. We wonder why such pain and suffering has come to our household. Everything was good just a few months ago. What went wrong? What did I do to bring this to us? However, there is no point in wondering why. Sometimes things just happen. Sometimes people get hurt. Sometimes people fall into depression. We wonder why these things have had to happen to us. Where in all of this is our Higher Power, our God? Why isn't anything happening on that front?

We can't change what happens to us, but we can work to understand it. With the help and support of our Higher Power, we can learn not to blame ourselves and we can help our depressed loved one overcome self-blame. We can be patient even though we don't understand why this illness is hurting us and someone we love.

Depression is a very common condition that strikes some people, through no fault of their own. It is uncommon, however, to find those people who are able to love and support one another through these difficult times, seeking to understand why there is no comfort or why someone they love has to suffer so much.

Higher Power, help me to reach out to those who seek
understanding of depression. Help me to love myself
and my depressed loved one through all of this.

We can help the depressed person to recognize that the new day is one in which he or she might show some signs of improvement. Whether we do that through getting them out of bed and the bedroom or simply by helping them respond to the alarm clock, it helps them to fight, no matter how small a fight, against the demon of depression.

Eating Your Broccoli

Issues of appetite often manifest themselves in depressed people. Whether they overeat or undereat, their health is at stake. Undereating causes the body to lose strength, to lose the ability to fight infection. When too much food is taken in, the body has to deal not only with the stress that is put upon it from depression, but also with the physical complications too much weight can bring—joint problems, heart difficulties, lung complications.

The "baby blues" had carried on for longer than Karen cared to admit. Her baby was past the two-month mark, and still Karen felt empty and had difficulty relating to her baby boy. She often would just feed him and then turn him over to her husband or her mother and go off to be by herself. She had also stopped eating much. She felt large and ugly and thought the only way she could get her old self back was to diet and lose the extra fat that had come with her pregnancy.

When Karen's husband, Ben, came home from work each day, he quickly discovered he was the only parent interested in making sure there was food in the house for the family, which included two other children. He was short on time and energy, so when he managed to run to the store, he filled the cart with fast and easy food but few fresh fruits and vegetables or whole grains. He and the kids had something to keep them fed, but Karen was wasting away to nothing. Ben soon realized that postpartum depression was present. With medication, Karen's mood and interest in the baby improved, but it was still a struggle to get her to eat. After consulting with their doctor, Ben finally recognized that healthy eating was one of the keys to helping his wife.

Capable adults can't be forced to eat, but they can be presented with good food. Make sure there is an adequate supply of fruits around for eating. Offer vegetables at every meal. Avoid sugars and too much processed food if at all possible. It's not possible in every situation to provide the best foods, but it is possible to choose the best from that which is available. An apple instead of applesauce. A baked potato instead of a processed potato mix. Fish instead of a marbled-fat steak. Help your depressed loved one by keeping the candy and other goodies out of the house. It will even help you as caregiver to approach the situation in a better light when you eat well also. In Karen's case, good food coupled with the right medication helped her to overcome the depression that had darkened her life and diminished her relationship with her child.

Tips for Daily Living

1. Accept your feeling that your loved one is different because of the depression. Keep in touch with how you are feeling and acknowledge your own feelings of anger, frustration, and sadness.

2. Return to the "C" of PACT and draw in your supportive community to help, even if only sporadically, or for small chores.

3. Don't expect everything to go right the first time. Just as dance steps take practice, so do the things we do to fight depression in our loved one.

4. Remember that not everyone understands depression. Accept people at the place where they are, and gently and regularly help them to gain new insight.

5. Don't overspend. If you are going on errands with a loved one, set an amount for spending. It will help with reining in impulse buys.

6. Take time for yourself. Plan things to do with friends, church members, or others that will take you out of the depression loop on a regular basis.

7. Learn to say no. Letting go of extra responsibilities will help tremendously in an already stressful situation.

8. Remember that an important part of health is good food—fresh fruits and vegetables and whole grains.

9. Take a small amount of time each day for yourself, whether that be a walk, a bubble bath, or whatever. You need that time to yourself to stay sane.

10. Don't be afraid to seek help from a therapist or other health professional if you find yourself sliding too close to the blackness of depression. It can happen, and staying on top of your feelings is the best way to prevent being swallowed up by them.

Exercise

The evidence is overwhelming: exercise in varying amounts boosts the endorphins that help to elevate mood. In addition, the right exercise can help us feel better and ready to deal with the struggles coming our way.

John had been a cross-country runner throughout his high school years and decided to pursue it during his college years. Circumstances prevented John from making the college team. Right around this time, he began to have difficulty with his studies. The people he used to hang around with in the cross-country group were now not around, too busy with the sport and too busy with their studies. Suddenly he no longer had anyone to talk to or bounce ideas off. As the days passed, he became more and more of a loner. He didn't run any longer, even for relaxation, and he found he was skipping his classes with increasing regularity. Soon John wasn't getting up in the mornings because there was nothing to get up for.

When his sister came to visit, she was surprised to find John in such a condition. One morning she dragged him out of bed and insisted he go running with her, claiming it was too dark out and she didn't know the area well enough to go alone. Reluctantly, John agreed, running with her for over three miles. When John was winded and sure that he couldn't go any farther, they stopped for some breakfast. John began to talk with his sister, the cloud having receded for a while. He was able to tell her all about things that had been going on in his life, and with her assistance, he began to seek help.

In John's case, the runner's endorphins kicking in after having been gone so long were what he needed to help him pause and look at what was happening to him. He was able to look at his situation, at least temporarily, in a different light, which gave his sister enough information to begin to seek help for him.

Brad had struggled with depression for eleven years. His wife, Liz, had helped him navigate those years, trying and discarding a long series of antidepressants. She helped get him to therapy appointments, but he'd never found just the right person to work with. Finally, when Brad tried a new type of antidepressant that had come onto the market, Liz began to notice that it did have a positive effect on his illness. Around the same time, he was referred to a therapist who helped him learn and follow through with strategies for overcoming the negative internal voices that kept him from functioning well. Depression had been a long, hard road that had taken a toll on their marriage, but things definitely looked better for Brad and Liz than they had for a long time.

Still, Brad struggled with exhaustion and with persistently "down" moods, and when Brad struggled, Liz was affected as well. It wasn't until his new therapist convinced Brad to make a point of walking for at least half an hour every day that they noticed unprecedented improvement. At first, Liz had to remind her husband every day to get out and get walking—after all, she had as much of a stake in his recovery as he did. After a few weeks of a consistent exercise routine, Brad seemed like a new person and Liz felt the man she had married so long ago had returned. Not long after that, he was able to face looking for a job for the first time in years. Daily exercise was the boost Brad needed to get over the final hill to recovery from depression, and he needed the loving support and constant reminders from someone who loved him to make it happen.

Endorphins are a powerful part of our bodies' makeup and have pain-relieving, mood-boosting properties. There are three types of endorphins, and one of these types is linked to exercise. These are called beta-endorphins and, according to studies, they appear to have the strongest effect on the brain and body during exercise. Endorphins can open the door to taking the steps that are necessary to deal with depression.

Errand Time

Running errands can prove to be quite challenging for a person living with a depressed individual. Whether you do errands together or the depressed person goes alone, unique situations present themselves. Sometimes the purpose of the errand will be forgotten entirely by the depressed person, with the result being that nothing is accomplished, sometimes with far-reaching consequences. Other times, the errand is done too thoroughly, with similar effects. If errands are done separately, there may be anger on the part of the caregiver when the depressed person fails to follow through, or comes back with more items than were needed. If errands are done as a couple, the caregiver may become frustrated at the slow pace at which the depressed partner moves.

Meena didn't know that George was depressed when they started living together. All of their friends thought of them as the perfect couple who had well-paying jobs, who were willing to try new things, and who were very much in love. All of that changed once Meena spent regular time with George. He slept until the last possible moment before heading off to work. When he would come home, he didn't want to do anything other than read the paper and go to bed early. When she expressed concern to her friends, they would laugh and say, "George? Depressed? You have got to be kidding." She thought it was "just her"; she was reading him wrong and just needed to get used to his habits.

One Saturday Meena decided she wanted George to join her for the weekly grocery shopping. She thought if he came along, they would purchase more of the foods he liked. It might even spark his diminishing appetite. Once inside the store, George couldn't decide on which shopping cart to use. Finally, after George selected and rejected seven of them, Meena just took one and started down the aisle, with George reluctantly following. She asked George to pick out some apples and a bunch of bananas, and she started to choose their vegetables. When she was done with her tasks, she realized George was not around. She looked back and spotted him at the apple section. She walked up to him and asked if he was finished. "No," he said, continuing to sort through the apples. Meena began to lose her temper. "Come on, George. We don't want to spend all day in the store. How about we choose some fish for tonight?" George just looked at her and said he had to get the apples. When Meena prodded him to move, George swung the bag of apples around and hit her in the side with it. Meena, shocked by his childish behavior, tried to get him to move on. "Come on, George, we need to go." Harsh, angry words followed. The outing and the day were ruined for both of them. Meena was too upset to spend much more time in the store, and they went home with only a small part of their grocery shopping done.

Reflections

- *What do I most enjoy about living with my loved one in spite of his or her depression?*

- *What behavior has been the hardest to accept?*

- *How can I respond to my loved one in a more positive way?*

- *What do I need to do for myself that would make daily life with my loved one better?*

Not every errand ends in such a way, but it is an illustration of how simple things become complicated in the life of a depressed person. When you love that person, it is difficult to understand and to work through what appears to be the simple task of carrying out errands. Depression does have a way of making it difficult for some individuals to prioritize, not to blow things out of proportion, or to carry out simple tasks. When we live with a depressed individual, we assume they have the ability to carry out these tasks and forget that their brains are not working in the same way as ours do.

Take time when it comes to errands. Check with your depressed loved one to make sure he or she feels comfortable in handling the errand. Go along with your loved one and stay engaged with what he or she is doing, offering suggestions as you go. Don't insist things go your way. Let him or her proceed at his or her own pace, and if you are concerned that what he or she is doing is dangerous or has the potential of escalating into a dangerous situation, come up with a distraction. Curb your annoyance or frustration if at all possible. Giving in to those feelings will only complicate the situation. Above all, start with small errands and gradually build up to larger ones as your loved one begins to feel more and more capable. Sometimes errands with your depressed loved one must wait until he or she is feeling better and is more capable of handling this part of daily life.

Try This

Take a moment to recall some of the most beautiful and healing things you know, whether a favorite piece of music, a baby's laughter, a garden of flowers in bloom, or a colorful sunrise. Consider the "why" of such beauty. Remember that for every ugliness in life that we don't understand, a Higher Power has given something beautiful to help us appreciate life around us.

Jobs and Finances

Many of us define ourselves by our jobs. What we do often translates to who we are. In a situation of depression, that identification can be even more pronounced. To begin with, a person with depression is probably not in line for the "Employee of the Month" parking spot—perhaps he or she is sleeping late or leaving work early, lacking concentration and consequently making an unacceptable number of mistakes, mistakes that wouldn't have happened had the depression not been present. When his or her job is lost, the person with depression can feel a complete loss of self-worth and of purpose. This doesn't even touch upon the fact that the lost income usually has a profound effect on the family.

Mike and Peter had both graduated with law degrees. Mike landed a job with the law firm he interned with and he had an offer from another firm as well. Peter was having a great deal of difficulty coming up with a position. The law firm that he had interned with hadn't made an offer, and no other offers were showing up. Mike tried to be as supportive as possible, but as the days went by, Peter was no longer going to job interviews or even sending out resumes. Mike, when he arrived home each day, found Peter lying on the couch and watching television, having done nothing in the way of looking for a job. Then one day Peter made the astonishing statement that he didn't love Mike anymore. Nothing had happened as far as Mike could see other than the lack of a job for Peter. However, things continued to get worse between them. Peter spent his days crying, and finally said he was going home to his parents and that the relationship with Mike was over.

Loss of job, change within that job, or the inability to get a job can be so much more complicated when a person is living under the cloud of depression. Clear thinking is not one of depression's hallmarks. The depressed individual might express the thought that he or she is not good for anything—or, like Peter, transfer the feelings into the relationship, carefully avoiding the pain of job loss or the inability to land a job by displacing those feelings onto a partner. The loss or the ongoing lack of a job can have giant repercussions for the family unit as well as for the unemployed family member. Suddenly, ability to pay the mortgage or buy food comes into question. How is someone living with the depressed person expected to cope?

Meditation

"If you want to feel rich, just count the things that money can't buy."

Anonymous

A glance at the checkbook tells you that the money is not going to stretch far enough this month. The feeling of shame that wells up in you when you buy food with food stamps tells you once again that things are not well in your household. A dress you'd love to buy but can't afford pounds home the point. All these things tell you again and again that the finances in your house are not good. Perhaps your partner can no longer work. Perhaps child care takes most of your salary. Perhaps neither one of you can find a job. Perhaps Social Security just doesn't make ends meet.

Often at times like these we move to the pity pot to sulk over the fact that it is poor, poor me who is having to put up with this loss of money, and we hold on tight to the fact that we are miserable.

Instead we need to let go (at least with one hand), and let God. We can look to what we do have. Is there a roof over our heads? Were we able to meet the bills this month? Are the children healthy? Am I able to take time for myself? We have to let go and trust God while we remember what it is that really makes us rich—the love of that Higher Power and the love of our family and friends. We can say "rich, rich me" instead of "poor, poor me" and find that that little mantra can help us through yet another difficult moment, letting us see a glimpse of the light at the end of our loved one's depression.

Help me to let go and let God, and
remember how rich I really am.

First, remind yourself and your partner, if necessary, that this too will pass and difficult times will not last forever. Second, don't be afraid to ask for help. Remember the "C" in PACT. The community is ready and willing to help you through this difficult patch. Many organizations can help with food, clothing, and even, in some circumstances, with figuring out how to pay a mortgage. On the following page is a listing of community resources to help with locating organizations, institutions, or programs that can be of help in your particular situation.

Third, if you need to seek financial help, be sure to remember that it is okay to do so—no matter what you were told when you were raised or what you have come to believe. Try not to be ashamed of the fact that you are in need. You are in need at present, but someday you may not be. When that day comes, perhaps your experience of being in need and asking for help may make you uniquely positioned to help others.

Turn to your Higher Power, and remember that with the help of your Higher Power and the help of your community you can overcome whatever difficulty comes your way.

Public Assistance Resources

Free and Reduced School Lunch Programs—The National School Lunch Program is provided by the United States Department of Agriculture. Qualification is based on income. For more information, contact your local school or visit the website:

www.fns.usda.gov/cnd/lunch/.

LIHEAP—The Low Income Home Energy Assistance Program helps low-income households meet their immediate home energy needs. For specific details, check with your state social service agency or your local utility company. For a general overview of the program, visit the website: www.acf.hhs.gov/programs/liheap.

Medicaid—Medicaid medical benefits are available in every state. Eligibility and benefit amounts vary widely. The website www.cms.hhs.gov/MedicaidGenInfo/ provides a general overview of Medicaid programs.

State Health Programs—Most states offer low-cost medical insurance programs for children whose families do not qualify for Medicaid. Check with your state social service agency for details. Your neighborhood school nurse may be able to provide you with information as well.

United Way 2-1-1—This simple telephone number and related website, www.211.org/, connects people to those who can provide help with food, housing, employment, health care, counseling, and other services in their communities.

WIC—The Special Supplemental Nutrition Program for Women, Infants, and Children provides federal grants to states for supplemental foods, health care referrals, and nutrition education for low-income pregnant, breast-feeding, and nonbreast-feeding postpartum women, and to infants and children up to age five who are found to be at nutritional risk. For information and to apply, visit the website: www.fns.usda.gov/wic/.

Relationships Outside the Circle of Depression

When depression descends on a household or partnership, it often causes the main participants to draw in on one another, withdrawing from friends and extended family, as they try to keep their struggles with the disease a secret.

Jeannette used to enjoy going to a quilting group in her neighborhood. It always meant a good time—lots of laughs, good food, and more knowledge about quilting. Lately, though, she has been avoiding the meetings. Ever since her husband, Gary, developed depression, she has found she is spending more of her time cleaning up the mess that follows in Gary's wake—a friendship that was broken when Gary lost his temper; a boss who is upset with his missing so much work; a doctor who keeps urging her to bring him in for an evaluation; his family, hurt because he no longer calls. She finds she has little time for anything else except the "great cover-up," as she calls it. She would be mortified if her mother or some of her good friends found out. They wouldn't understand that Gary is sick. They would talk and drop snide remarks, and she's sure they would eventually stop calling. She reflects that most of them have stopped calling already—and they don't even know for sure what's going on.

> **"People usually consider walking on water or in thin air a miracle. But I think the real miracle is not to walk either on water or in thin air, but to walk on earth. Every day we are engaged in a miracle which we don't even recognize: a blue sky, white clouds, green leaves, the black, curious eyes of a child—our own two eyes. All is a miracle."**
>
> Thich Nhat Hanh[*]

---

[*] *The Miracle of Mindfulness* by Thich Nhat Hanh, Copyright © 1975 by Thich Nhat Hanh. Reprinted by permission of Beacon Press, Boston.

Whenever we try to conceal depression, or keep it a secret, we become sicker. We allow ourselves to be pulled in by one of its tentacles, and we walk a fine line between falling into the pit and keeping a precarious balance. One of the best things you can do for yourself and your partner is to let people know about the depression, to keep it a secret no longer. Light sheds understanding and love on any situation.

Of course, we need to be careful with whom we share our story. We all know people who do not know how to keep boundaries, or who do not respect the individuals in a situation, but instead like to pass on the latest "gossip" to whoever comes along. Consider carefully before sharing your information. Some people will get very little of the story—only enough information to let them understand what is happening. Others will get the whole story and generally will step up to the plate to help out in whatever way they can. They will be the ones supporting you in prayer and action, who will be willing to help when you need some time away. They will be the ones you can turn to in a crisis situation. Remember the "T" in PACT. Truth will help us cope with anything that comes our way, especially when we let in those who will love, support, and dance with us through the darkness.

Alone in a Crowd

In spite of our best efforts to reach out, no matter what books and articles we read in order to learn more about this devastating disease, sometimes our best efforts fall short. Perhaps those we look to for assistance are caught in a crisis of their own. Perhaps we just wake up one day and feel that no one really understands, or our depressed loved one has even distanced him- or herself from us. We feel alone and bereft. To make matters worse, a lot of people won't have a clue what we're dealing with, and we can have a very hard time helping them to understand.

If you find yourself feeling alone even among others, one thing that might help is to find a way to completely stay outside the arena of depression. Remember Liz, whose husband Brad had suffered from depression for over a decade? Liz was very familiar with the feeling of being alone in a crowd. Though everyone they knew was aware of Brad's illness—ten years is a long time to try to hide that big a problem—she didn't feel she could keep talking to people about it. It was an old, tired subject, one that for a long time seemed to have no solution. So over the years she learned to keep her pain to herself. She knew it probably wasn't the healthiest route, but it was the easiest by default.

Then one day Liz happened to be thumbing through a catalog of continuing education classes from the local community college. She ran across a description of a jewelry-making class and, on a whim, she decided to enroll. It turned out to be a sort of accidental lifesaver, as Liz put it. Spending an hour a week with strangers who knew nothing about her life was a relief—it gave her a place to forget and just be one of the other students. She could join in a casual conversation without fearing that someone would bring up the eternal question, "How's Brad doing?" And she was doing something with her hands, using her creativity.

This kind of escape can make a big difference in our ability to jump back into the fray of life with depression. Getting away can have the same effect as putting a bandage on a toddler's scraped knee. If we don't look at the sore place, the pain goes away for a time. Of course, we have to be careful not to lose touch with our reality—we still have to keep up with our responsibilities and we have to make an effort to keep ourselves healthy physically and emotionally. Finding a group in which we can take on a different persona, in which we don't feel alone in the crowd, can be a temporary way to cope.

When we are going through these lonely times, it's also time to pay some close attention to our own daily actions and routines, independent of the depressed person. Perhaps we've stopped doing the little things each day that keep us going. It could be we're still doing these little things but we're so tired and frustrated that we are not enjoying them anymore. Some daily attention to self-care is definitely in order. For a detailed discussion of self-care, take a look at Chapter Seven—Self-Care to Fight the Darkness.

There is no magic potion for dealing with these feelings. The best we can do is allow ourselves to feel them, to acknowledge that they are temporary, to find ways to care for ourselves while they are occurring, and to remind ourselves that we have our Higher Power, who will not forget us.

When we feel stronger, we can reach out—to our depressed loved one, to those who have supported us but who may now need our help, and even to those who do not understand. It is only in outreach that we are able to heal, to grow beyond ourselves, to love another. An anonymous author once wrote that "life might not be the party we hoped for, but while we're here we should dance." Let's join hands with our depressed loved one and those who are trying to understand and dance together so that our love and care can brighten the darkness for us and for everyone facing this deadly darkness.

> **"When we are alone on a starlit night, when by chance we see the migrating birds in autumn descending on a grove of junipers to rest and eat; when we see children in a moment when they are really children, when we know love in our own hearts; or when, like the Japanese poet, Basho, we hear an old frog land in a quiet pond with a solitary splash—at such times the awakening, the turning inside out of all values, the 'newness,' the emptiness and the purity of vision that make themselves evident, all these provide a glimpse of the cosmic dance."**

Thomas Merton*

---

* *Thomas Merton's Paradise Journey: Writings on Contemplation* by Thomas Merton, Copyright © 2000 by Continuum International Publishing Group. Used with permission.

CHAPTER SIX

Parenting Blindfolded

"Let parents bequeath to their children not riches, but the spirit of reverence."

Plato

Parenting comes in many forms. Most familiar is the traditional parenting situation—two adult parents or a single adult parent, with offspring. Sometimes parenting is extended when there's a second marriage and two families are blended. Everyone at some time has either had a parent or been a parent, or both. Those of us who have taken on the role know all too well that it's a difficult job. There is no book, seminar, or course that can fully prepare us, or cover all the curveballs aimed at parents.

Then there's a very different type of parenting—the kind that comes up from behind, puts its hands over our eyes, and commands us to "guess who you're parenting now?" And we realize it could be anyone we know asking the question—our own now-elderly parent, our spouse, even a friend or a sibling. When depression strikes, it can take away the victim's ability to function normally as we would expect an adult to do. In this case, we can find ourselves acting out the role of parent in a way we never expected. We might end up parenting an adult child we thought was out of the nest, our own parent, someone recently bereaved, a sibling getting over a divorce, a friend—even a spouse or partner. This is a type of parenting that catches us unaware and unprepared, just like the "blindfold-guess-who" greeting. It takes time to figure out just what's going on, and what we're expected to do.

Many Faces of Parenting

When we are dancing through life when depression is present, parental responsibilities look very different than we expected. Let's look at some of the parental roles in which we might find ourselves:

- Jamel is nine years old and has lately been very irritable. He was always a very easygoing child, and this irritability is a change his mother noticed immediately. In addition, he no longer enjoys building models, which at one time had been his greatest area of interest. He had always had lots of friends, and one particularly good friend, Shawn, who shared Jamel's passion for model building. Jamel no longer invites Shawn over, and spends a good part of the day complaining that there is nothing to do. When his mother suggests building models with Shawn, Jamel erupts in anger and ends up being sent to his room. His mom is at her wits' end trying to figure out what's wrong and what she should do.

- Paul and Diane had been married for fifteen years when Paul's depression hit. Suddenly Paul was like a little kid, unable to make decisions or run errands, without a job, and given to sudden crying outbursts and strange, inappropriate behavior. He had to be told where to go and when to do different things or they would never be done. Diane found herself taking more and more responsibility for running the household—from paying bills to caring for their four children. Now, with the depression, she realized she was parenting a fifth child.

- Joanne and Dave had been planning on taking their two teenagers on a vacation to the Rockies. Fifteen-year-old Tom was excited about the trip and quickly joined in the planning. Tara, seventeen, was indifferent. She showed no interest in the plans and harped on everything that could go wrong on the trip. When, following a long-standing family tradition, she was assigned a portion of the trip to plan, she seemed unable to concentrate on the task and couldn't decide on what sites they would see and where they would stay. As the trip drew nearer, Tara started to complain about aches and pains, sure that she wasn't well enough to go.

- When Jane came home with her new baby, she didn't realize that she would now have two children to care for—the new baby girl and her own husband. Darrin found excuses for not holding the baby or meeting any of her feeding, bathing, or changing needs. He found it difficult to sing or make eye contact with the baby, and when Jane approached him to discuss the problem, he flew into a rage, insisting nothing was wrong. Soon he was sleeping a lot, he lost interest in sex, and he cried at the drop of a hat. Jane became very concerned when Darrin casually mentioned that he wondered how the baby would react if he put a pin into the baby's soft spot.

- Wendy's father was seventy-six and she was always proud to point out that he was active, involved, and happy. One day, though, she arrived at his apartment to pick him up to babysit her children and found him sitting on the couch in his underwear. The house reeked of urine and the sink was full of dirty dishes. When she asked him what was wrong, he said that he just didn't feel like doing anything. By the time he got up each day, it was almost dark. Why were the days so short, he plaintively asked his daughter as he reached for a bag of potato chips on the floor by his chair. Wendy did a double-take as she realized that her father must have put on ten pounds or more since she last saw him—only last week.

- Lyle's partner, Andrew, did a great job of keeping the household running by paying the bills, shopping, taking care of the cooking and cleaning. When that changed overnight, Lyle didn't know what to think. Lyle, who had been working very long hours, came home one evening to find the electricity and gas turned off, and Andrew asked for the fifth time in a week if they could go out to eat. Finally, Lyle realized nothing had been done around the house in some time. Bills were unpaid, the kitchen shelves were empty, and the trash cans were overflowing.

Traditional parenting is never easy. Parenting is even more of a challenge when it doesn't fall into the traditional setup, when we suddenly find ourselves parent to a friend, parent to a parent, parent to a spouse. The presence of depression can mean that we have to step up into the role of guiding our loved one, much as a parent would guide a young child through a playground maze.

"Hug me."

All Children, Everywhere

How Traditional Parenting Can Change

Very young children

Perhaps one of the most difficult situations surrounding depression occurs when children are involved. When one of the traditional caregivers is laid low with depression, it can make for some very difficult challenges for the other parent. Not only must he or she take care of the person dealing with depression, but he or she must do the everyday parenting of the children, effectively acting as a single parent to a child *and* parenting an adult. It's a difficult, easily overwhelming task.

First, the children need to be told, in age-appropriate terms, what is going on. Sometimes we feel we need to spare children from the difficulties of life when it is much kinder to let them know what the situation is and answer all their questions as best we can. Not discussing the presence of depression in the family with them can result in their blaming themselves for having caused the illness.

For babies and toddlers, of course, communication will not be so much verbal, but during this time you can be liberal with your hugs and kisses and laughter. Let them know they are loved and will be cared for. Spend time with them; by doing so you will realize you are renewing yourself. Remember those endorphins? Hugs, like exercise, release endorphins that can serve to lift our mood.

For young children, explain in simple language what is happening and why. Be sure to let them know that it is not their fault and be sure to share those hugs and kisses and laughs with them. You might say, "Daddy is sick with an illness that has nothing to do with you. It is not catchy. It doesn't mean that he doesn't love you. This illness is why he's been so grumpy and sleeping all the time." Reassure them that things will get better. "Daddy will be visiting some doctors who will help him get better and help him seem more like himself. This illness won't last forever."

"Tweens"

For older children, be more definitive in your explanation. They'll have more cognitive ability to deal with some details. Discuss why depression happens and how it can be dealt with. Reassure even these more worldly children that it is not their fault. They still can feel they are capable of causing the disease through an argument, a shouted angry response, or even an unspoken thought. It is often older children who pick up on the tension and stress in the household, and consequently take sides.

Sometimes, without parents meaning for it to happen, older children are used as an emotional buffer by either parent. It's vital at this time to maintain boundaries—you're the parent, with the bulk of the responsibility, and they must be allowed to be children. Don't let them become your new best friends during the depression of your loved one. Yes, you need someone close to you to unload on, but that person needs to be another healthy adult. Children are not emotionally ready to handle being our "friends." Draw boundaries and try your best to keep them.

Teenagers

One conversation we must have with teens when they have a depressed parent is the possibility that they, too, are susceptible to depression. These kids are old enough to know about the genetic component to the illness, and they need to be on the alert for the illness in their own lives. Share with them the symptoms they should watch for, and let them know you'll be watching as well, for the sake of their own health. No need to frighten them.

Depression is not necessarily their destiny. Just help them become aware and let them know you'll be there for them at all times, no matter what.

Teens living with a depressed parent can have additional issues to deal with. Because the nondepressed parent so often feels overwhelmed and in need of a break, the older teen might be the one turned to for help: babysitting, shopping, or taking the depressed parent to the doctor. This is all well and good *occasionally*, but not all of the time. Teens still need time to goof off and have fun with friends. Make sure to allow for that. Above all, speak to your teen about what is happening in the family. Be aboveboard with them about the depression and encourage them to ask questions. Let them know you are willing to talk about it with them at any time.

We have a tendency, when kids get into their teens, to ignore their needs for physical touch. Hugs often go by the boards, and we keep a physical distance. But when teens are living with a depressed parent they may need even more physical expressions of love than ever. Show tangible expressions of love, whether that is a handshake, a pat on the back, or a quick hug on the way out the door; and don't forget to use words to express your love, whether that is a shouted "I love you" as they head to school or "Be careful" as they go off with friends. Let them know they are of value and loved very much.

Children away from home

Even when children head off to college or to jobs in a different city, they are still part of the family and need to be kept informed of the family's health and well-being. When a spouse is suffering from depression, children need to be kept informed of how their parent is doing. If not, when the children return home, they will be facing turmoil to find the lifestyle of the family changed due to depression. Honesty is paramount no matter the age of the child.

Reflections

- *What effects might this time of depression be having on our children?*

- *What words can I use to help our children understand what's happening?*

- *How can I express love and caring to help our children feel secure during this time, both verbally and physically?*

"Making the decision to have a child is momentous. It is to decide forever to have your heart go walking around outside your body."

Elizabeth Stone

When a Child Is Depressed

Younger children

Childhood is supposed to be a time of innocence and happiness, of tree-climbing and daydreaming. It's not supposed to be a time of depression, yet it happens in many families. Kids get depressed. What is a parent to do?

We know depression affects the way people are able to function, or do their jobs. So first of all, look for the red flags in the jobs children have—going to school and learning, spending time with friends, and interacting with the family. If a child begins to lose interest in school or seeing friends, it could signal that something is happening. Children can manifest depression through a lack of interest in play, a change in sleep, or declining grades at school. A self-assured child suddenly becomes clingy and begins to experience meltdowns when a parent is leaving for work or a night out. Kids who are potty-trained may begin having "accidents" during the day, while other kids may complain of physical aches and pains. All of these signs tell you, the parent, that it is time for an evaluation. Start with your pediatrician or family doctor. The doctor can determine if any physical reasons are behind the changes in behavior. If there is no physical cause, the doctor will be able to refer you to a psychiatrist or psychologist who deals with children.

If it turns out that the child is experiencing depression, it is important that help be sought as soon as possible. Waiting can complicate the illness. One of the treatments frequently chosen for children is psychotherapy, either on its own or in combination with medication. Therapy allows the child to learn ways to manage symptoms. Learning these strategies can keep the disease from spiraling out of control and causing difficulties that could have long-reaching effects.

The use of medication, especially for younger children, is still under study. There are, however, some medications that are considered safe. Using "off-label" medications (the use of medication for conditions for which they weren't intended) and the use of adult medications for children are both to be avoided. Talk with your doctor and research current trends on medication for children, should the suggestion arise. Any medication has the potential to make the depression worse instead of better. Careful monitoring of medication is necessary. Check with the Mayo Clinic or other reputable sites for the latest on the pros and cons of antidepressant medication for children.

The involvement of the family is critical. When the parents learn coping strategies they are better able to offer their child the time, warmth, and caring that are vital to the treatment of the disease in children. Research has shown that extra time spent with children, so they can feel safe and loved by parents or caregivers, makes a significant difference in the treatment and overcoming of depression.

Remember, parents are the primary advocates for the child. A child generally does not request therapy. Listen to your child's feelings, assuring him or her of your support—and then follow through, immediately.

Meditation

*"Parents can only give good advice or put them
on the right paths. But the final forming of a
person's character lies in their own hands."*

Anne Frank*

With the anticipated arrival of a child, whether through birth or adoption, we catch ourselves wondering what the child will be like. What kind of laugh will he or she have? Will she be dynamic and active, enjoying sports? Will he be contemplative, and enjoy sitting and reading before bed? What kind of personality will he or she have? So many questions are never really answered. We are in fact getting to know another human being from scratch. Wondrous as it sounds, it is not always an easy road. As the days go by and you learn more and more about this person, you find yourself worrying about his welfare, wondering if she will get over her cold, wanting to protect him at all costs. In short, this little being has won your heart without even trying, and you would be willing to do anything to keep that person well and happy.

Our ability to love and care for another is a real gift. We are able to intertwine our hearts with theirs, and yet we have to keep those two hearts separate. We can teach, we can lead, we can offer, we can assist, but we cannot make this other person do anything he or she doesn't want to do. Sometimes those choices cause happiness and sometimes they cause heartache. We can't control those choices, but we can offer our undying love and support and keep that heart walking in the world.

Let me allow my heart to be always open to love.

---

* Used with permission by Anne Frank Fonds, Basel, Switzerland.

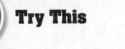

Try This

Take a few minutes to bask in the love you have for your child. Think back on all your child has learned from you. Congratulate yourself for doing a good job in these areas.

Teenagers

As you watch for signs of depression, teenagers present a different challenge than do younger children, poised as they are between childhood and adulthood. It can be difficult to know from day to day exactly where we stand with them. The moodiness and testing of boundaries common in the teenage years can throw an extra wrench into the works when depression is a concern. Keys to parenting teens through this darkness include knowing the individual child, going out of our way to stay in touch and maintain a loving relationship, and keeping ourselves informed about how depression can affect teens.

Symptoms of Depression in Teens

- Agitation, restlessness, and irritability

- Appetite changes (usually a loss of appetite but sometimes an increase)

- Difficulty concentrating

- Difficulty making decisions

- Episodes of memory loss

- Fatigue

- Feelings of worthlessness, hopelessness, sadness, or self-hatred

- Loss of interest or pleasure in activities that were once fun

- Thinking or talking about suicide or death

- Trouble sleeping, excessive sleeping, or daytime sleepiness

- Changes in behavior or in school activities may be depression symptoms, even if no "down" mood is noticeable:

  - Acting-out behaviors (missing curfews, unusual defiance)

  - Criminal behavior, such as shoplifting

  - Faltering school performance, grades dropping

  - Highly irresponsible behavior pattern

  - Use of alcohol or other illegal substances

  - Withdrawal from family and friends, spending more time alone

If such symptoms are present consistently for two weeks or more, the possibility of depression should be explored and treatment should be sought.

National Institute of Health[1]

Columbia University offers new research that finds nearly 50 percent of teens suffer from some form of depression, anxiety, or other psychiatric disorder. While the number may seem staggering, remember that it points to the fact that adolescence is a difficult time in our society. Mild anxiety or depression may be temporary. This is why it's so important to check in regularly with your teen, keeping a finger on their emotional pulse and letting them know you are available and interested.

Reflections

- *What changes have I seen in my child's behavior that could indicate a deeper problem?*

- *What other adults can I check in with who could provide helpful insight into my child's current behavior and moods?*

- *Where can I go for resources and referrals within our community for dealing with childhood depression?*

Full-fledged depression will last for weeks or months or even longer, impairing the ability of the depressed individual to participate in normal day-to-day life. It may be overlooked as parents and teachers write depression symptoms off as unhappiness or "moodiness" typical for the age, blaming hormones and other factors. Consequently, many teens go undiagnosed and untreated.

Suicide is increasingly prevalent among gay, lesbian, bisexual, and transgendered teens. The "It Gets Better Project," initiated by syndicated columnist and author Dan Savage, offers hope to these teens whose life experiences have been so difficult that they see no way out other than taking their own lives. Through more than 10,000 user-created YouTube™ videos, LGBT and straight adults (including many celebrities and President Barack Obama) remind teens in the LGBT community that they are not alone, that there are many people who support and care for them, and that their lives definitely will get better once they make it through their teenage years. Visit www.itgetsbetter.org to learn more.

Being aware of risk factors is vital. Sometimes stressful events, such as an unexpected divorce or an unwelcome move, can trigger depression. Other times the illness comes on with no warning or identifiable cause. Parents should be aware of certain risk factors, including stress of schoolwork or schedules, loss of a loved family member, or loss of friends. Teens who suffer from attention, learning, or behavioral disorders are more susceptible to the illness. Family history of depression increases the risk. Girls tend to have a higher incidence of depression than boys.

During a time of emotional turmoil, you might become aware of experimentation with drugs, alcohol, or sex. Risk taking or hostile behavior may also be present, according to the National Mental Health Association. Swift treatment for depression in teens is crucial, not only to stem these dangerous behaviors, but also to head off the possibility of suicide, the third leading cause of death for Americans aged ten to twenty-four.

Warning Signs That a Teenager Is Contemplating Suicide

- Feelings of hopelessness or worthlessness, depressed mood, poor self-esteem, or guilt

- Not wanting to participate in family or social activities

- Changes in sleeping and eating patterns: too much or too little

- Feelings of anger, rage, need for revenge

- Feeling exhausted most of the time

- Trouble with concentration, problems academically or socially in school

- Feeling listless, irritable

- Regular and frequent crying

- Not taking care of him- or herself

- Reckless, impulsive behaviors

- Frequent physical symptoms such as headaches or stomachaches

National Institute of Mental Health, 2011[2]

When parents suspect the presence of depression in a teen, listening is key. For example, if a teen repeatedly and over time complains of feeling "down," parents should be on the alert and ready to intervene. There have been cases in which a teen has requested counseling to no avail; parents sometimes refuse to admit to a problem and hope or assume it will just go away on its own. But any request for such help must be taken seriously. Sweeping potential problems under the rug is a dangerous course of action.

When it's time to look for help for a potentially depressed teen, there are places to turn. Getting the input of trusted school personnel or other adults who know the child can help create a clearer picture of what's going on. Parents of the teen's friends or youth leaders at your house of faith can provide valuable information as well. School counselors can help with referrals to therapists or other resources. Don't be afraid to look to those who have more information.

All teens experience ups and downs. Fights with a friend or parent, feeling the need to "fit in," worries over a failed test, bad grades, an unsuccessful audition or tryout—all these and more can challenge the emotional stability of a teenager and lead to normal feelings of sadness or grief. Usually these episodes are brief, unlike depression, which is intense and prolonged. Parents in this situation must be watchful, arming themselves with information and with assistance from other trusted adults and medical professionals, before depression takes over.

Depression at any age is a nightmare. When teenagers, already caught in the confusion of changing hormones and the onrush of new thoughts and feelings, suffer from the disease, they need all the help they can get in order to dance through depression into the light. Be their dance partner by being ever-alert, ever-honest, and ever-loving.

Postpartum Parenting

The birth of a baby is expected to be a joyous time. New life should bring smiles and happiness, along with the feeling that we, as parents, have the power to help this young person grow and succeed. We anticipate, making plans and just enjoying the lifelong journey with our children.

Unfortunately, not everyone experiences these positive reactions to a new child. According to the National Institute of Mental Health, hormonal and physical changes, along with the responsibility of caring for another human being, make women susceptible to depression after giving birth. Many women experience a brief episode of "baby blues," but 10 to 15 percent of women experience a more serious depressive episode within a month of giving birth. Women are at a higher risk if they have a history of depression symptoms, a high level of stress, or a lack of a supportive circle of friends and relatives.

However, it is not only women who suffer from this type of depression. More recently, studies have been focused on the father's depression, also known as "paternity blues," which can occur in the first three months following the birth of a child. Feelings range from inadequacy to frustration related to the new paternal role. Often the father chooses to have little if any contact with the child. When the mother is depressed, it can lead to a greater risk of depression for the father as well.

Symptoms of "Baby Blues" and Postpartum Depression

Signs and symptoms of the baby blues, which last only a few days or weeks, may include:

- Mood swings

- Anxiety

- Sadness

- Irritability

- Crying

- Decreased concentration

- Trouble sleeping

Symptoms of postpartum depression are more intense and last longer than those of the baby blues. These more aggressive symptoms may include:

- Loss of appetite

- Insomnia

- Intense irritability and anger

- Overwhelming fatigue

- Loss of interest in sex

- Lack of joy in life

- Feelings of shame, guilt, or inadequacy

- Severe mood swings

- Difficulty bonding with the baby

- Withdrawal from family and friends

- Thoughts of harming oneself or the baby

If untreated, postpartum depression may last for a year or more.

Mayo Clinic[3]

When postpartum depression strikes, the nondepressed parent is faced with what seems like an impossible load of responsibilities. We all know the stress of caring for a baby is exhausting in itself. When almost all the care for the baby falls to one healthy parent, and at the same time that healthy parent must care for, encourage, and help find treatment for their depressed spouse, it can be more than one person can handle.

Enlisting the help of a supportive community—the "C" of PACT—is a true lifeline in this case. Friends and family are likely to be more than willing to assist with baby care so the nondepressed mother or father can catch up on rest. They can jump in to help with shopping and meals. They can provide rides to the many medical appointments that must be kept, both for the new baby and for the depressed parent. All the support they will have wanted to give anyway will be doubly precious when postpartum depression darkens the experience of parenthood. If you have no close friends or family nearby for whatever reason, consider becoming involved in a neighborhood group or a faith community that might come to serve as a support line. Such a move can also enrich your lives in the future as you return to health. Support groups specifically for parents living through postpartum depression are available. Check for one in your area. (See sidebar, page 99.)

It can be especially difficult for a new parent to admit to the presence of depression. When life looks vastly different from the soft-focus, rosy glow of a diaper commercial, we feel we've failed. Guilt can creep in, as we wonder why we can't be exclusively joy-filled about the new life in our midst. In spite of such feelings, truth—the "T" of PACT—must be kept front and center. More than one life may be on the line if we don't confront postpartum depression head-on and enlist as much assistance as possible. Depressed new parents can suffer health crises or face suicide. Children of parents suffering from postpartum depression can experience health issues and developmental delays. Sharing truth with our depressed loved one, our supportive community, and our Higher Power can make all the difference in keeping everyone healthy.

Effects of Postpartum Depression on Parenting

The following are some of the ways parental depression may affect parenting:

- Being less responsive to the baby's needs

- Feeling out-of-sync, withdrawn or being unable to play with the baby

- Avoiding of the child and/or partner

- Providing inconsistent or intrusive parenting

- Showing little positive emotion toward the child, such as smiling

- Showing more irritability or even aggression

- Having difficulty knowing how to best soothe the baby

Adapted from *This Emotional Life*, a production of the Public Broadcasting System[4]

When a parent suffers from postpartum depression, help must be sought as soon as possible in order to head off declining health for both parent and baby. If your partner is showing symptoms, let him or her know you're concerned and are willing and able to help. Talk to your doctor about medication that would be safe for the mother and the baby or for the father. Discuss a course of treatment that might make a difference. Take advantage of support groups in your community. If you can, arrange for someone to come and help with the child care, housework, and other chores, allowing both parents to have some time for themselves for rest, recharging, and any medical appointments that might be necessary.

ℹ Resources for Postpartum Depression Information and Support

Postpartum Support International—www.postpartum.net/

This website offers links to local support groups, as well as helpful information.

National Alliance on Mental Illness—www.nami.org

NAMI's website provides links to local support resources, especially for families and friends of those with mental illnesses.

Online PPD Support Group—www.ppdsupportpage.com/

This site offers online discussion, informational brochures in multiple languages, and a number of other resources.

Helpguide.org—www.helpguide.org/mental/postpartum_depression.htm

Look here for accurate, up-to-date information about baby blues and postpartum depression.

Postpartum depression, if left untreated, can mushroom into deeper depression and can severely endanger both mother and child. Seek the help and support you need, whether you are the one suffering or the one called in to parent both the baby and the adult. Recent research shows that a child can change quickly for the better when a mother or father recovers.

Though relatively rare, postpartum psychosis is another illness that can affect new mothers. This condition, which may appear suddenly on its own or develop out of postpartum depression, causes the mother to lose touch with reality. Sufferers hear voices and commonly experience irrational guilt. If help for the condition is not found, mothers with postpartum psychosis may attempt to harm themselves or others. Should symptoms be noticed, immediate medical attention is required.

The Effects of Parental Depression on Infant, Toddler, and Child Development

Parental depression affects children in many ways, mostly in the area of parent-child attachment.

Infants may display the following behavioral changes:
- Disrupted sleep and eating
- Fussiness and difficulty accepting soothing
- More frequent illnesses
- Lack of or less frequent vocalizations
- Slowed language development
- Less exploration
- Fewer "social smiles"

Toddlers may display the following changes in behavior:
- Increased number and duration of tantrums
- Irritability
- A frowning/angry face
- Limited ability to self-soothe
- Heightened level of frustration
- Cognitive, fine motor, and speech delay
- Less social interest and exploration
- Social withdrawal from adults and peer playmates

Preschool-age children may display the following behavioral changes:
- Reduced vocabulary
- Increased speech problems
- Higher rates of developmental delays
- Classroom behavior problems

Handbook for Early Head Start Staff Working with Depressed Parents[5]

When the Child Becomes the Parent

We don't expect to have to take on a parental role with our own parents. After all, they've been the ones who have guided us through life, who have taught us so much. However, with a greater aging population and with a shift in how we take care of our elderly, more and more children are finding themselves taking care of their parents. Some assist their parents as they struggle through a physical illness or declining health. Others have to grapple with their parents' suffering from the disease of depression. Trying to parent our own parent makes dancing during depression a challenging proposition.

Unfortunately, not everyone has a good relationship or history with his or her parents. Should this be the case, consider carefully whether you are the right person to take over the responsibility of helping the parent through his or her depression. You might not be, and that is all right. If, however, there is no choice, you must have a plan of action for keeping yourself healthy during the time you are caring for your parent. Without that plan you can find yourself quickly spiraling into depression yourself because of past history and present danger.

> **"We never know the love of a parent till
> we become parents ourselves."**
>
> Henry Ward Beecher

Of the six million Americans over the age of sixty-five, one in three suffers from some type of depression. Whether due to side effects of medication, a difficult physical challenge, or dealing with the fallout of aging—loss of a spouse or close friends, loss of independence, living with chronic pain, living alone—depression can rob an older person of dignity.

The best thing a caregiver who is parenting a parent can do is to respect the parent. Let him or her know you are helping as friend-to-friend, not as child-to-parent or parent-to-child. This respect will go a long way in maintaining a comfortable relationship. An attitude of respect will also help elicit responses to necessary questions, and in getting cooperation with medical treatment. It's easy to become impatient or irritated, expecting aging parents to act as they did when they were younger and in better health. Giving way to frustration, however, can destroy trust and make interactions more and more difficult. Try to acknowledge that both of you are slipping into unfamiliar and possibly unwelcome roles. Further, work to accept the changes you see in your parent. Look for positives and laugh over the oddities that go along with aging.

Try This

Be prepared for frustrating circumstances when trying to parent a parent. When anticipating a visit, a trip to the doctor, or some other interaction with a depressed parent, stock up on mental diversions you can use to help both of you get through the experience with good humor. When tempted to toss out words of frustration, imagine how your favorite book or movie character would react. If conversation becomes unproductive or unpleasant, have a juvenile knock-knock joke up your sleeve that you can pull out to relieve the tension. Divert a litany of complaints by relating something funny you saw at the grocery store. Even if your efforts don't seem to have a positive effect on your loved one, you may keep yourself amused enough to keep going.

Reflections

- *How would I characterize my lifelong relationship with my parent? How has it changed?*

- *What are my true feelings about taking on a parenting role for my parent? Who can I talk to if these feelings are hard to manage?*

- *How has depression changed my parent's personality? What does this mean for me?*

- *Who can share some of the parenting responsibilities in this situation?*

Depression in the parent of an adult can bring out relationship issues that other depression situations do not. Our parents, as we know if we have children ourselves, are accustomed to being the protectors and caregivers—and we're accustomed to being the beneficiaries of that protection and care. When we trade places, strong emotions can overtake us as we get used to "a new normal."

Older people dealing with depression may not say anything about it, or they may not even recognize a problem. We have to remember that open and frank discussion of depression—or any mental illness—is a relatively new societal concept. The older our parents are, the less comfortable they're likely to feel in admitting to a problem. Older generations were expected to "pull themselves up by their own bootstraps." Depression, for them, was a shameful weakness. We can try to change this mind-set through honest discussion and education, but we're not always able to overcome a lifetime of bias. If depression is suspected in an older person, you might consider that person's primary care physician as a starting point for treatment. A trusted doctor may be able to make some headway in framing the conversation about depression in terms that are easier to accept.

Any depressed person will need help monitoring medications and moods, but a parent living alone is even more in need of such help; check on him or her regularly. Encourage regular healthy meals, whether by assisting with shopping or looking into some of the offerings available to senior citizens such as Meals on Wheels. In every instance of help, treating the older individual with respect and patience is the most loving thing you can do as a friend and "parent."

Of course, as with any situation when we're caring for a depressed person, we have to pay attention to our own needs. Because we're dealing with what seems like the loss of the person who has been a guide and support all our lives long, we're likely to have a hard time coping with this "parenting" relationship. There will be times when we simply don't have the energy— emotional or physical—to do the check-ins, to drive to an appointment, to follow up on the medications. Consider carefully who can stand in for you. Your siblings, other relatives, neighbors, or church friends may be able to offer some relief when you need a break. Consider splitting duties—one person to monitor medications, a few people to provide transportation, several people to assist occasionally with meals. A team, or community, working together might be able to provide better care than one person alone.

"Parenting" a Depressed Senior

- Invite your loved one to go places with you or join them in going to do something they want to do.

- If possible, schedule regular activities for them and assist if they need help in planning or in getting to a place. Being around others often helps depressed individuals to feel better.

- Help them plan and prepare healthy meals, or if that is not possible, brainstorm with them ways in which healthy meals can be a part of their lives.

- Use your best skills to encourage the senior to follow through on treatment. With anyone who is depressed, failing to follow through on treatment often means a deeper plunge into depression.

- Talk with your loved ones about ways in which medication can be taken regularly and help in whatever way possible for that to become a reality.

- As with anyone battling depression, watch for suicide warning signs and seek professional help immediately if such signs are present.

Helping an older loved one—a parent, an aunt, or a friend—is not always easy. In our culture, which tends to devalue the elderly, we need to do what we can to help seniors feel valued. Checking in often, staying for a chat, helping with transportation will not only make them feel valued, but you may feel better as well. Above all, value each senior as a person, a person who just happens to be struggling with depression but who, with love and support and respect, can deal with it and come back into the light.

Parenting a Spouse or Partner

Parenting a spouse is a difficult situation. We are used to sharing the joys and sorrows of life together and instead, depression has lowered your loved one's level of functioning until it seems to match that of a child. Loss of decision-making skills, inability to maintain a routine, turning inward—these traits can look very childlike. When we see them in someone we've come to depend on as a life partner, they can seem childish and selfish. Before we know it, we go from being equal partners to being, effectively, a parent and child.

This problem can be even more pronounced as a depressed spouse or partner enters into treatment. The healthy partner is called upon to make and follow through with appointments, to monitor medications and their side effects and effectiveness, to help the person remember to eat healthily and exercise. Soon we forget what it was like to work, live, and love side by side with the person we planned to spend our lives with; we're too busy providing parental-type care.

In this situation, it's essential that we look to alternate sources for affirmation of our own value, a gift the one person we've chosen to walk through life with is no longer able to provide. Remaining in contact with our Higher Power is a good place to begin. The same Higher Power who lovingly created us can be a source of affirmation in the dark times of life when we feel lost and alone. Reaching inside ourselves for affirmation is important as well. Spending time with friends and loved ones outside the circle of depression can help us keep dancing, reminding us of what is good and healthy and whole about us—and also help us reenergize so we can go back to our depressed partner and keep trying to maintain a relationship that will still be there when the light returns.

Try This

When acting as a parent to your life partner, hurt and frustration can become the standard. Battle these feelings with the healing power of music. Perk yourself up with upbeat songs that lighten a down mood. Give yourself permission to shed a few tears as you listen to a more mellow or haunting piece. Recall better times with music the two of you listened to before the time of depression. Good music can express emotions we're incapable of fully sharing, and can give us a soul-nourishing boost when we need it the most.

Taking on the role of a parent to our partner can do some fairly significant damage to a relationship. Resentment can grow quickly on both sides, and when depression begins to lift, the relationship patterns that were adopted for survival can be hard to shed. Professional counseling can go a long way in ensuring that the relationship is able to able to continue to grow and remain healthy. Once the depressed person has begun to stabilize, consider looking for referrals to a good marriage/couples' counselor who can help you learn new steps to an old dance.

Traits of Good Parenting

When you become the one who must parent others, how do you survive? Here are some traits that might help during the difficult time of parenting another.

1. **Listen and Communicate**

   When you find yourself in a situation in which you unexpectedly have to act as a parent, communicating and listening are perhaps the two greatest skills needed. Stress the importance of sharing needs and concerns openly and clearly, as well as listening to others' needs and concerns fully. Many times we talk but fail to listen. Intentionally pause to hear what people are saying as if for the very first time. Repeat back what you heard in order to clarify. Share your needs openly and honestly. Model these communication skills and expect others to do the same. Listen to the nonverbal things that are communicated: tone of voice, sighing, body language, and so on. Good listening enables us to turn the kaleidoscope and respond in an authentic rather than a perfunctory way.

2. **Affirm and Support**

   Affirmation, the "A" of PACT, is necessary when we're parenting a depressed person. Receiving support and encouragement for our own abilities and traits can help us survive the experience. If we don't get that affirmation from the sources we've looked to in the past, we can go to other friends and family—and certainly to our Higher Power. In addition, be clear, firm, and consistent regarding what you expect in terms of behavior, responsibilities, and any other areas that affect you both. Be very clear about how far you are willing to go and what you will not accept. Ask for the same from others. It's the best way to affirm and support one another.

3. **Respect and Trust**

   We all want to be treated with respect. When we don't yell at a child when they spill their milk, when we respond with patience and kind words to a difficult, hurting parent, we cultivate a respectful relationship that affirms, supports, and opens the door for listening and communication. Model trustworthiness by promising only what you can truly deliver. Follow through with what you've started. Expect the same from others.

4. **Don't Be a Martyr**

   Even in the darkest time, those suffering from depression can be asked to share responsibility, whether it is for taking their medication as scheduled or to report to loved ones if things are going wrong or right. Sharing responsibility can lead to a dance toward health and keep you from being a martyr. Make your peace with the fact that you have chosen to be the giver in this relationship during this challenging time. Yes, you may spend a great deal of your time doing things for this person. But it's your choice. Don't take it personally if you don't get much in return. Look for affirmation and appreciation elsewhere, in nondestructive ways, of course, when you don't get it from the person you're caring for.

5. **Keep a Sense of Humor**

   Almost every situation has a lighter side, if we look hard enough. Distance yourself enough that you can find something at least a tiny bit amusing. Allow everyone in the situation to have fun and laugh—that's what makes life worth living.

6. **Keep to Routines and Celebrations**

   Routine is a lifesaver in times of depression. Routine creates a comfort level that helps us know that life will go on. The bedtime rituals, the birthday traditions, the regular sound of the alarm; all these help us to stay grounded and to remember that there are still good, normal times to be had.

7. **Keep in Touch with a Higher Power**

   It is important to stay in touch throughout the day with our Higher Power, no matter how that Higher Power manifests itself. That regular contact enables us to stay rooted in what is right and good and helpful to us as we deal with depression.

8. **Make Sure to Have Some Fun**

When someone is depressed, we forget that we can relax together. Too often we get caught up in the intensity of depression and forget to give ourselves permission to have fun. Activities that help us forget about the depression for a time can make all the difference in the outlooks of everyone involved.

9. **Seek Help When Needed**

Reaching out for help when problems overwhelm us can be very hard to do, but a good parent is willing to accept help for the good of his or her child, and in this case for the good of the relationship or the family. When we recognize our need for others to help us through the darkness of depression, we open the door to health and healing.

Parenting, even under ideal circumstances, is a rough ride. When you add depression into the mix, when someone you never thought you'd parent becomes your charge, it becomes as complicated as trying to navigate a maze wearing a blindfold. When we take off the blindfold and "parent" with trust and confidence, with our Higher Power's help, our changed relationship can survive and grow.

CHAPTER SIX NOTES

1. National Institutes of Health. 2010. *Adolescent depression* [Online]. Available from http://www.nlm.nih.gov/medlineplus/ency/article/001518.htm (accessed 6 August 2010).

2. National Institute of Mental Health. 2011. *Suicide: A major, preventable mental health problem* [Online]. Available from http://www.nimh.nih.gov/health/publications/suicide-a-major-preventable-mental-health-problem-fact-sheet/teen-suicide.pdf (accessed 22 July 2011).

3. Mayo Clinic Staff. 2010. *Postpartum depression* [Online]. Available from http://www.mayoclinic.com/health/postpartum-depression/DS00546/DSECTION=symptoms (accessed 4 March 2011).

4. The Public Broadcasting System. 2011. *Parenting and PPMB; First Contacts Last a Lifetime* [Online]. Available from http://www.pbs.org/thisemotionallife/topic/postpartum/parenting-ppmd (accessed 4 March 2011).

5. "Alumbrando el camino/Bright Moments: A Curriculum for Staff Working with EHS Parents with Depressive Symptoms DHHS;" Administration for Children and Families, University-Early Head Start Partnership Grant Number: 90YF0056/01 Principal Investigator: Linda S. Beeber PhD, PMHCNS-BC University of North Carolina at Chapel Hill, School of Nursing Chapel Hill NC 27599-7460

CHAPTER SEVEN

Self-Care to Fight the Darkness

"Self-love, my liege, is not so vile a sin as self-neglecting."

William Shakespeare

here is a fundamental truth we must embrace if we're to survive the depression of a loved one: it is not selfish to take care of oneself. Just as a flight attendant instructs us to put our own oxygen mask on first in case of an emergency, we have to be healthy and whole ourselves in order to have anything left to help the person we love out of the darkness of depression.

But self-care doesn't always come naturally. Many of us have been told from childhood to think of others first, to put our own needs and wants at the end of the list. Though service to others is a worthy endeavor, we sometimes do it to the point of neglecting ourselves, for fear of being labeled "selfish." Neglect of our own needs is a dangerous proposition, especially for a caregiver of a depressed person. Truth be told, if we've taken on the responsibility of caring for a person who is depressed, surely "selfish" is the last adjective that could be used to describe us.

At the same time, we have to recognize that caring for a depressed person may be beyond us. If we're physically ailing, if our own emotional state is precarious, or if we are overwhelmed by other difficult circumstances, taking responsibility for the ongoing care and support of someone else might be unwise. In such a case, focusing on a depressed person's needs while ignoring our own problems can lead to disaster, and can mean doing a great disservice to the person we want to help. This is a good time to recall the "T" in our PACT with our Higher Power. Being honest with ourselves and with our Higher Power about the truth of our own situation is vital, for the sake of everyone involved.

"In dealing with those who are undergoing great suffering, if you feel demoralized and exhausted, it is best, for the sake of everyone, to withdraw and restore yourself. The point is to have a long-term perspective."

Adapted from teachings of the Buddha

We must remember that self-care might mean NOT being the one to care for a depressed person. Self-care might mean turning care over from the beginning to someone better situated to handle the issues associated with depression. It might mean entering into the caregiver relationship for a time, but knowing when to pass the baton. In the end, though, self-care will always mean that we keep in touch with our own needs in order to do the best we can for the one we love.

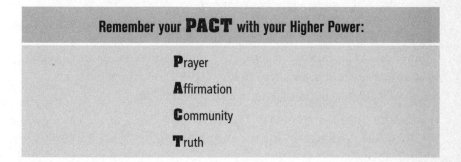

Remember your **PACT** with your Higher Power:

Prayer

Affirmation

Community

Truth

What Does Self-Care Look Like? Recall Your PACT

A review of PACT is the first thing to do when considering self-care. Our PACT can be the foundation of our survival.

We need connection with our Higher Power through prayer. When we have this relationship to fall back on, we receive support, a sounding board, and a wholeness we tend to lose when we try to stumble through the darkness under our own power.

Affirmation from our Higher Power and from friends and family is always vital, but perhaps never more than when a person we love, who would ordinarily provide us with positive regard and affirmation, is depressed. When we look for and recognize the love others give us for simply being who we are, we can gain the strength we need to keep going and keep dancing.

We need a community around us. Depression can detract from the friendship, good times, and support we once received from a loved one. Reaching out to a community of friends at church, in our neighborhoods, in our social circles, and in our families gives us someone to laugh with, someone to pick up the kids from school when we're delayed, someone to listen when we're reaching the breaking point. A community does all this for us, and we can do the same in return when we are stronger.

Truth can be a lifeline during a period of depression. It may be our natural instinct to hide the painful details, to downplay how bad things really are. But the more we hide our problems, the more frightening they become. Buddha said, "Three things cannot be long hidden: the sun, the moon, and the truth." When we try to hide the truth, it will eventually come spilling out in ways and at times we may regret. Speaking the truth can free us of our burdens, and can in turn lead to support and affirmation from our community; we can begin a continuous cycle of healing.

Meditation

"Loneliness is the first thing which
God's eye named, not good."

John Milton

Depression is an illness of loneliness. Depressed people feel
that no one can possibly understand how they're feeling;
they're isolated in their pain. We feel we can't share the
frustration and worry of caring for a depressed person;
we're isolated by our experience.

We were created for community—the community of
the Higher Power who wants to be in relationship with
us in both the light and the darkness of our lives; the
community of others who can walk with us on our journey,
supporting us, loving us, affirming us so we can keep going.
In community is wholeness and wellness, a strength we
lose in isolation.

Higher Power, keep reminding me of the steadfast
relationship you have with me, and the relationships
with others with which I've been blessed.

Try This

Make a list, mental or written, of people who have been a part of your supportive community. Look through old photos to remind you of friends you've lost touch with. The list and photos themselves can help dispel feelings of isolation. Now reach out to one of these people with a phone call, a note, or an email. Before the week is out, make a date with one of them so that you'll have a plan for being part of a loving, caring "we," an essential part of wellness.

Physical Health

Most of us are aware of what we need to do to stay healthy. Whether we do what we know we should do is another question. Even when life is going well, busy-ness and bad habits can keep us from a routine that promotes good physical health. When we're dealing with the depression of a loved one, our own physical health is much too easy to neglect.

It can be tough to maintain healthy choices and normal routines in the face of an illness that does its best to destroy routine and normality. Our schedules get interrupted by crises or by doctor and therapy appointments. Our time gets eaten up in listening to and encouraging the depressed person. We may be tempted to dash into a fast-food drive-through because we didn't have time to get to the grocery store. We're so worn out that the thought of exercise seems impossible.

But this is when we need to go out of our way to be more conscious of the preciousness of our time and of the choices we make, for the sake of staying healthy ourselves. Keep up with physicals and screenings. Avoid unhealthy food. Only schedule activities if they will allow you to get sufficient sleep. Make time for exercise—the same endorphins that will help a depressed person feel better will help keep you in a positive frame of mind as well.

Simple Actions for Daily Physical Health

Following are a few tips for keeping up with healthy habits when you find your routine disrupted and your energy sapped:

- Spend a few minutes with your calendar each week. Block out a time each week when you can hit the grocery store for healthy foods that are quick and simple to prepare for a snack or a small meal.

- While you've got your calendar open, check on when you're due for your next annual exam, lab tests, or any other regularly scheduled doctor visits. Keep up with these appointments as a preventative measure—heading off poor health is a lot easier than recovering from it.

- Make a point to eat a meal together as a family several times a week. Our definitions of "meal" and "family" may vary widely, but sitting down together for healthy food and talking time with those we love has proven to be a key step for maintaining health.

- Be on the lookout for creative ways to sneak in a little exercise. Deliberately park as far from the door of your destination as possible. Take the stairs instead of the elevator. Dance while folding the laundry. The same endorphins that elevate mood for depressed people can do us a lot of good as well.

- Get plenty of sleep. If late-night discussions with the depressed person are often keeping you up, create a rule about timetables for conversation, for example, "no soul-searching after nine p.m." Though his or her sleep patterns may be disturbed, yours need to be stable, and you may have to be the one to set limits.

- Give yourself permission to take naps. According to the National Sleep Foundation, twenty-to thirty-minute naps improve alertness without creating grogginess or interfering with sleep at night.

Emotional Health

Though depression is not viral or bacterial, those of us who have been close to depressed people know the illness can be contagious. When someone we care about goes around with a sorrowful countenance, our own face begins to mimic that sad look. When they focus constantly on the negative or lash out in irritation, these moody episodes infect us, too. As Ralph Waldo Emerson put it, "We become what we think about all day long." Just as we must keep an eye on our physical health, we have to monitor and protect our emotional health when we're spending a great deal of time and energy with a depressed person.

Emotional Health: Be Alert for Signs of Depression

By now, you're probably pretty familiar with the list of depression symptoms. What you might not be considering, though, is whether that list applies to you. It's easy to be so focused on the person we're concerned about that we miss similar depression-related symptoms in ourselves. The more time we spend with a depressed person, the more likely we are to start experiencing some of those symptoms.

Be very deliberate about finding someone you can trust to talk to openly during this time. Not only do you need someone to whom you can let go of all the frustrations, worries, and fears; you also need someone who is capable of sharing good times with you. Whoever this person is, provide him or her with a complete list of depression symptoms, and ask him or her to help you monitor your moods, if you think he or she would be likely to catch something you might miss.

Consider keeping a journal of your own moods and thoughts. Make a point of writing down your feelings as well as a quick rundown of your activities every day or two. If you feel you don't have much time to journal, keep it to a short list of words that summarize how you felt and what you did. Review your entries every week or so. Such a record can be very valuable in keeping track, over time, of the major trends in your own moods and abilities. If you notice consistently over time that the words you use are negative, or that what you're able to accomplish day-to-day has taken a sharp downturn, it could be a sign depression is sneaking up on you. In this case, it's time to take another look at the list of common depression symptoms and see where you stand. If necessary, seek out a professional who can help you assess your emotional state and make recommendations for your own treatment, as needed.

In short, for your own sake, be alert for signs of a downturn in your own mental health. Don't allow yourself to become "collateral damage" in the war against depression.

Emotional Health: Creating Healthy Boundaries

We ache to see our loved one dealing with sorrow, confusion, and crisis. It's natural to want to jump in and help wherever we are needed. But dropping our own lives every time others call can wear us out and create other problems we'll have to deal with later. Setting and maintaining boundaries can be essential for self-care and even for survival.

We need to deliberately create occasions that enable us to distance, or at least detach, ourselves emotionally from our depressed loved one. A bit of time away to be ourselves again in a healthy environment, out of the circle of depression, can be necessary if we're to keep helping in the long term. Take some time to read a book, go to a movie, or talk with a friend. Whatever is relaxing and rejuvenating, that's what you need to do at every opportunity. Take a very intentional "vacation" from the stress of dealing with depression. If there's concern about the loved one's safety and health during our self-imposed "time-outs," we might enlist the help of a trusted friend or family member who can check in and monitor in our place.

We might also find it necessary to choose not to step in during some depression-created crises. Repeatedly rescuing the depressed person has several negative results. It allows him or her to remain in a needy state instead of learning to handle life independently again. Then, too, jumping to the rescue wears us down in frustration and anger.

But creating boundaries when someone we care for is in great need is easier to say than to do. Creating scripts ahead of time for use when the need arises can make circumstances go a little more smoothly. Picture a likely scenario based on past experience with your depressed loved one. What words might you be able to say that would express love and caring while also calmly stating your own need for space? Here's a sample script between "Sharon" and her depressed sister, "Denise," that could be used when Denise phones with an alarming issue:

Sharon: "I'm really glad you feel safe turning to me when you need help. I hope you know I care about you and want the best for you."

Denise: "I do know that. I really depend on you."

Sharon: "I'm glad I'm able to help you. Right now, though, I need you to know I'm worn out and need a little time to myself."

Denise: "Oh, I'm so sorry. I don't mean to wear you out. I just mess everything up."

Sharon: "You don't mess things up, honey. And you don't wear me out. It's just the situation that's difficult. The depression you're dealing with affects me, too. Will you let me help you think of a way to get through this current issue without me? I promise I'm not disappearing on you."

Denise: "Okay. I'm not sure I can work through this without you, though."

Sharon: "I know you can. Let's think of some actions you can take to relax and feel better until you've got this problem resolved. And let's think of someone you could spend some time with to take your mind off all this stuff for a while."

Of course, we have to keep in mind that conversations rarely go as smoothly in reality as they do in our minds. But imagined and rehearsed scripts can help us feel prepared, and help us stay strong in the face of the temptation to jump in and rescue.

Reflections

- *Under what circumstances might it be appropriate for me to step away and allow myself some space?*

- *What can I do to keep track of my own emotional state during this time?*

- *What kind of activities might help me relax and reenergize during this stressful time? When will I make time to do some of these things?*

- *What carefully chosen words might I use to relate my concern while still maintaining healthy boundaries?*

Emotional Health: Maintain "Normal"

Again, life with a depressed person seems anything but normal. Daily life is disrupted with emergencies, crying jags, and emotional upheaval. Social life can evaporate as the depressed person becomes unwilling or unable to spend time with friends. The laughter, camaraderie, and mutual support we've come to enjoy disappear. Before long, we might forget what normal even looks like.

Deliberately keeping up with our own regular routines can go a long way in helping us maintain some semblance of normal life. If going to the gym several times a week has been a habit in the past, make it absolutely sacrosanct now. Keep those movie dates with friends. Read the paper in the morning over a cup of coffee. Watch your favorite TV show. Don't allow someone else's inability to keep up with daily life send your own routine into a nosedive.

Emotional Health: Keeping a Sense of Humor

Life is funny. It just is. A sign posted on a street corner advertising both DNA testing and tax preparation from the same source? Worth a laugh even on a bad day. When the darkness of depression throws a shadow over our lives, we have to go out of our way to seek the humor in life. It's there if only we take the time to look for it.

Look up a few comedy movies or TV shows. End the day with at least a brief viewing as often as possible. Read a collection of your favorite comics. Get a CD of a comedian's routine and listen to it on the drive to work. Do something silly and mindless with the kids—blow bubbles, put on a dance show in the living room, color in a coloring book. Whatever makes you laugh or helps you see the lighter side of life, seek it out and escape for a time.

Even in the pain of depression, humor can shine through. One family discovered that the antidepressant medication taken by their depressed father caused him not only to talk but to invent funny poems and songs in his sleep, delivering a nightly performance that kept them laughing. If humor is an instinct we've ever had even to a tiny degree, it's something we need to cultivate now, of all times. If we don't keep laughing, we'll surely be reduced to crying.

> **"We should consider every day lost in which we have not danced at least once. And we should call every truth false which was not accompanied by at least one laugh."**
>
> Friedrich Nietzsche

CHAPTER EIGHT

My Higher Power Is Hiding in the Dark

"Where love is, there God is also."

Leo Tolstoy

It's a fact, plain and simple: Depression takes a great toll on relationships. It robs its sufferers of the ability to look outward and to share and to listen. The illness does its best to break friendship, to harm marriage or partnership, to alienate family members. No relationship comes out of a time of depression without being changed. This change can, in the end, be for the better, but one thing's for sure: it will be a long, hard road getting there. It takes an almost superhuman effort to bring that relationship back into the light.

Ironically, there's another relationship that is put under tremendous strain, a relationship that could help us through the maze of depression: our relationship with our Higher Power. If you've experienced a life of faith, you know staying in touch with your Higher Power in the good times of life is a considerable challenge. Maintaining that relationship in dark times can seem impossible.

Where Has My Higher Power Gone?

Reliance on a Higher Power is a source of daily comfort for many. No matter what you call that presence—Yahweh, Allah, God, Source, Spirit, Vishnu—it is the journey of a lifetime to grow closer in understanding and learning. Through whatever spiritual practices we find meaningful, we seek to find a way through this life alongside our Higher Power. Prayer, study of holy texts, community with others of faith, worship—all of these and more aid us in our walk of faith. For those who do not believe in a spiritual power, striving for a spirit of goodness or truth may be a guiding principle that provides meaning and purpose in life. It is simply in our nature, as human beings, to look toward something bigger than ourselves.

Whatever form our Higher Power takes, it is a light in the twisting, turning shadows of life. We turn to our Higher Power for help in discerning the right path to take in our lives. We thank our Higher Power for the many blessings we receive, and we work alongside each other as we strive to understand our calling in the world. We petition the Higher Power in our concern for others or for ourselves, and we cry out to this Being when the darkest times of life threaten.

But it is in the darkest of times when we are likely to feel the loss of this presence. This Being who has created, loved, and affirmed us very often seems absent when times are hardest. We cry out, and in our despair we hear only a dull silence that echoes and underscores the pain we feel. Many who have lived with depression in a loved one have found that the devastating effect of the illness made them feel entirely cut off from their Higher Power.

Why Is My Higher Power Silent?

Overwhelming emotions are a hallmark of depression. The depressed person is awash in sorrow, despair, fear, anger toward him- or herself and toward life. The caregiver, watching this excruciating array of feelings, is easily overwhelmed by them as well. Who can stand by and see someone they love struggle so without hurting? Combine this bottomless well of pain with the work of coordinating treatment, taking over duties the depressed person once had, juggling finances, and any number of other aspects of our lives into which depression intrudes, and the result can't be good. If we're not very diligent in caring for ourselves in these circumstances, exhaustion is inevitable.

When we reach a state of exhaustion, many of our lifelines fly out the window. We're too tired to exercise. We're too tired to call friends. We're too tired to make the effort to eat healthily. We might be too tired to even think about any practices we might once have engaged in for staying close to our Higher Power. Anyone who's that tired is easily inundated by a wide range of emotions, and the number one emotion that reigns is a feeling of abandonment. The depression of the person we love makes us feel he or she has abandoned us. After all, depression's gripping focus has left nothing for conversation, support, or friendship. It doesn't take long for a feeling of abandonment to grow. If we don't share the truth with our community of friends and family, we feel they've abandoned us, too, even if it was our own decision to withdraw. If we become consumed with the difficulties of life as a caregiver, we risk losing contact with our God—and soon we feel our Higher Power has abandoned us as well. It's like a snowball rolling down a hill of dirt, picking up more and more ugly debris as it goes.

It's no surprise that the next emotion likely to come to the fore is anger. Yes, we know the person we love is suffering from a debilitating illness, but we still don't understand how he or she could turn from us so fully. Anger at what feels like betrayal is natural. Then, too, others who have been part of our support system are unlikely to truly understand how difficult things are, even if we are able to be truthful with them. This lack of understanding creates more anger. Our Higher Power, to whom we've cried out repeatedly, seems silent as our loved one continues to suffer, as we continue to suffer, as our anger grows.

But we've been taught that anger is a destructive emotion. We worry about lashing out in anger at the depressed person, thereby causing more hurt to one who is already hurting. We may think we can't afford to show anger toward the very community that is trying to support us, or that it's somehow cosmically wrong to be angry at God, and so we feel guilty for the mere fact of having such feelings, and next, we feel afraid of what might happen to us for having all these feelings. But these thoughts and worries are not necessarily accurate; we must accept ourselves and all of our feelings, and be kind, not only to our loved one, but to ourselves as well.

"Hatred and anger are powerless when met with kindness."

Author Unknown

Yet another aspect of life with a depressed person serves to disconnect us from the relationship with a Higher Power that we so miss. If we are the main caregiver for a depressed person, then as we move into the mode of "parent," huge responsibilities shift onto our plate. We become accustomed to being the one in charge—setting the appointments, making the decisions, handling the crises. We can't or don't trust the depressed person to follow through with much, so we slip into an overfunctioning mode in an attempt to hold things together. Soon we become so used to handling things on our own that we forget we're not actually alone—that our Higher Power is nearby to be a source of strength. We become so consumed with self-sufficiency that we can lose the inclination to turn to Someone we're pretty sure isn't listening or caring anymore, anyway.

It's a downward cycle of negative thoughts and emotions. When our thoughts and feelings become so consistently negative, it's all but impossible to see the light that our Higher Power holds out for us. We lose contact and can't feel God's presence. The light has been turned out on us, and we have no idea how to go forward.

Reflections

- *How has this time of depression affected my ability to connect with my Higher Power?*

- *What emotions am I experiencing that I could share with my Higher Power? How might such sharing help me stay in contact?*

Meditation

"What has been long neglected cannot be restored immediately. Fruit falls from the tree when it is ripe. The way cannot be forced."

The Buddha

Sadly, sometimes our relationship with our Higher Power is neglected when we are dealing with a loved one's depression. We spend our time railing against the heavens, wanting our prayers to be heard and answered, wanting things to be better, wondering "Why me?" The more we rant, the more convinced we become that things will not get better. We get angry at our loved one, and resent people who are unencumbered by the complexities of depression. As we rant, we also plant seeds of doubt that we water with self-pitying tears, until they threaten to take over the garden of our peace of mind.

Instead, we need to make the decision to plant the seeds of compassion and love. When we tend the seeds of love and compassion, we choke out the weeds of anger and resentment, and gradually our world comes alive. The friends and neighbors who have been there all along are "suddenly" there for us and for our family—because we've noticed that growth of love. The obstacles that have seemed like impenetrable walls are suddenly only hills that can be crossed hand in hand with a friend. Planting the seeds of love and compassion helps us to open our eyes to the ripe fruit of support around us. The type of garden we want is up to us. Weeds or flowers? What will it be?

Wondrous Master Gardener, help me to recognize the seeds of love and compassion already growing in my life. Give me the tools to cultivate them in my heart.

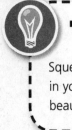

Try This

Squeeze out enough time to go for a walk, either in your garden or in a park. Even in winter there is beauty to see. Soak it in.

Reconnecting with Your Higher Power

As we've already discussed, we must be very intentional during this time of depression to take care of ourselves physically and emotionally. It's equally important that we deliberately care for our spiritual lives whether or not we've valued a relationship with our Higher Power in the past. Losing closeness with our Higher Power means losing out on an ever-present source of strength, comfort, affirmation, and love. When we've already lost so much—time, energy, a relationship with our depressed loved one—this loss is even more wounding.

So how, exactly, do we manage to hold on to our Higher Power in the darkness of depression?

- **Let go of guilt.**
  A sense of unworthiness or indebtedness is a common foundational belief of many traditional religious faiths. Nothing I can ever do, the thinking goes, can make me worthy of the love of my God. I'll never be good enough. Especially now, when depression has taken away my ability to reach out to God, when I've railed in anger at God's absence in my life, why would my Higher Power continue to care for me?

This kind of mental self-flagellation must be released before we can move on to continue and grow in our relationship with our Higher Power. At a time when our energy is at a low point, we definitely don't have any extra energy to waste on guilt. A God who is worthy of our adoration and worship is not a God who would turn from us merely because we're in too much pain to pray.

Try This

Dumping guilt isn't easy, but it's absolutely necessary. Practice letting go of this debilitating emotion. Determine at least three times throughout your day when you can spend five minutes repeating to yourself words such as these: "I am doing my best in a very bad situation. God loves me and stands beside me even when I feel I've failed." If you're able to manage it, try to be alone and still, eyes closed, while you repeat this affirmation. Picture the arms of your Higher Power around you, holding you close through what you perceive as your inadequacy.

- **Be in supportive community.**

  Our Higher Power created us for community. We need to be with others now, more than ever. Sometimes we need to be with people who can listen to our hurts and frustrations, with whom we can share our despair and our sense of being cut off from our Higher Power. Other times we need to be with people who can help us laugh and forget, who know when it's not a good time to ask, "So how are you handling the depression lately?" If we can express our bad times and our good times with people who care about us, we can be reenergized to approach our Higher Power with a more whole and healthy spirit.

- **Share your truth.**

  Be intentional about remembering that the "T" of PACT—truth—lifts a burden that's too heavy to carry. How can we seek help if we're not honest with ourselves about the way things are? How can our friends support us if they don't know what we need? How can we remain close to God if we keep the worst of our pain and suffering to ourselves? Without truth, we can't. Remember, it's not a sign of weakness to admit we can't go it alone. Our Higher Power never intended for us to be alone, and honesty with others and with God will help us reach a place of strength and comfort.

Letting go of guilt, accepting the support of community, and sharing our truth are important steps to finding our way back to the light of relationship with our Higher Power. But there's a fourth step we need if we're going to get to that light: intentional communication with our Higher Power through prayer, meditation, or whatever practice is common to your faith.

Praying in the Dark

How can I pray when I've lost so much? How can I pray when the object of my prayers is so silent, so distant, so absent? I barely have the time or energy to fall into bed each night—how can I possibly pray? These are valid questions, arising from the exhausting emotions depression throws at us. The answer to these questions lies in another question: what is prayer?

Many of us have been taught exactly what communication with a Higher Power is supposed to look like, how it sounds, when we are to do it, and what words we should use. If we don't follow these rules, we feel we've failed. During this time of depression, when we're struggling with a sense of abandonment, with anger, with faith itself, we must let go of these preconceptions and learn to embrace a new model of prayer. For the sake of spiritual health, consider this definition of prayer:

Prayer: Any thought, action, or imagery that allows me to express my true self to my Higher Power and/or to hear and feel what my Higher Power has to express to me.

We were each created as unique individuals. We each have varying strengths, interests, personalities. When we remember that these differences are a conscious choice of the Power who created us, we can allow ourselves the latitude to communicate with that God in whatever way feels most comfortable and most fulfilling.

Reframing our idea of what prayer is, acknowledging that our own personal style of prayer is holy and acceptable to the One who created us, can free us from a sense of inadequacy as we approach our Higher Power.

"The fewer the words, the better the prayer."
———
Martin Luther

Try This

Choose a daily time over the next three days when you can spend five to ten minutes in a new type of prayer. In the first minute or so of this time, deliberately clear your mind of words. Instead, picture a person, a place, or an object that stands for what is most on your mind and in your heart at this time. With eyes closed, focus solely on this image. Allow yourself to feel the ideas and emotions evoked, without trying to put them into words. Let these ideas and emotions fill your heart, and picture them entering the consciousness of your Higher Power. Allow this time away from the organizational structure of language to become a silent prayer.

When Prayer Feels Unanswered

Jill and Ryan had been married several years when depression took over Ryan's life. In a few short months he went from being an active, fulfilled man to being jobless and joyless, in the depths of the illness. That change was hard enough to take. What was even harder was the fact that no treatments—and they tried many medications and a number of therapists—made a dent in his depression.

Jill had spent her lifetime studying the teachings of her faith, and maintained a routine of prayer and meditation that kept her relationship with her Higher Power strong. She knew that both pouring out her heart and intentional listening were equally important in this relationship. But as Ryan's illness dragged on, and as Jill cried out to her Higher Power in desperation for healing, she was stunned to realize that she heard nothing in return. The God who had always been there for her now seemed entirely

absent. In anger and frustration, Jill gave up her lifelong practice of prayer and meditation. God obviously didn't care any longer.

It was two years later, when a new combination of medications and therapy finally resulted in a long-term improvement in Ryan's condition, that Jill found the ability to reflect on the barren time she'd experienced with her Higher Power. In hindsight she was able to see the sustenance she'd received from friends and family in the darkest times. She recognized the strength their marriage had gained in coming through the depression together. After a time, she came to acknowledge that these experiences were, in fact, evidence of the presence of her Higher Power. That power had simply been speaking in a language and with an answer she had not been able to understand until she gained the perspective of time.

Intentional communication with a Higher Power is a valuable aspect of survival when depression intrudes in our lives. Still, as we've discussed, it can be difficult to keep those lines of communication open. It's easy to become hurt and angry at what we experience as silence or abandonment.

Picture yourself at a locked door, and the key you hold in your hand—the one that is supposed to let you in—wasn't cut very well. You know from past experience that if you keep putting that key into the lock, keep jiggling it, keep turning it, the doorknob will eventually turn and you'll be able to open the door. You have to make many, many tries before you discover the correct sequence of jiggles and turns that makes the door actually open, but in the end, open it will.

Attempts at prayer can feel this way. What can be extremely difficult to remember—in fact, what we don't understand until we're standing on the other side of the door and the difficult times are behind us—is that all those attempts we made did serve a purpose. Each time we put in the key, each time we jiggled it around, we were learning something in the process, and progress was made.

Meditation

"The function of prayer is not to influence God, but rather to change the nature of the one who prays."

Søren Kierkegaard

When heartfelt cries to a Higher Power don't have the result we desire, it's natural to come to the conclusion that those prayers have gone unanswered. Perhaps it's a function of our instant-gratification culture that when our prayer requests aren't granted quickly, we assume failure. Often we hear someone say, *"I prayed, but my prayers weren't answered."*

What if, instead, we understood these possibilities?

"I prayed for healing and my Higher Power said, 'Wait.'"

"I prayed for improvement and my Higher Power said, 'Take some time for yourself.'"

"I prayed for a miracle and my Higher Power said, 'Appreciate small victories.'"

Just as our definition of prayer needs expanding, perhaps our definition of answer to prayer needs to grow. If we can understand that our Higher Power may have other plans for us than what we would ask for, we may feel less cut off from that Being when what we desire doesn't materialize on our own timetable.

Help me accept the answers you give me when I cry out to you, whether or not I understand them.

Reflections

- *What spiritual practices have been helpful for me in my relationship with my Higher Power?*

- *How might I manage to return in some way to these practices?*

- *How might my understanding of prayer and answer to prayer affect my ability to be in communication with my Higher Power?*

My Higher Power Is Different

Interpretations of a Higher Power are, fittingly, as different as the people making the interpretations. For those involved in religious traditions, that Higher Power might take the shape of Jesus, or Yahweh, or Allah. For some who have a deep faith but cherish no religious tradition, that Higher Power might be a Force of Energy that permeates their lives. For still others with no religious background, the Higher Power becomes a form of Truth or Beauty or Goodness with a lifelong journey of self-exploration and growth. No one's version of a Higher Power is better than another. Whoever or whatever that Higher Power is for you, the Higher Power has the strength, energy, and love to pull you up and love you no matter what happens. If your Higher Power is different from that of your neighbors, your friends, or your depressed loved one, it doesn't negate the power of the One who can help us.

No matter who or what your Higher Power is, carving out time for reflection, meditation, centering, and/or self-care is extremely important. Whatever it is that creates in you a sense of peace, of accomplishment, of growth, that is what you must strive to appreciate and attend to during this difficult time.

Allow yourself to devote the necessary time and energy it takes to nurture the Higher Power in your life. Reread a book that has had depth and meaning for you. Listen to music that creates peace and joy in your soul. Spend time in nature, absorbing sustenance from the earth and its beauty. Visit an art museum to drink in the truth and beauty of artistic expression. Use these kinds of experiences to help restore your balance and recall what is most important to you. Let these moments remind you of the Higher Power in your life, the Higher Power that says it is not an act of selfishness to care for the inner self. It is a necessary act of survival.

The person we were created to be can become lost in our attempts to care for someone who is depressed. As you experience the storm of emotions that accompanies the illness, allow yourself the space to be honest about what these emotions are doing to your spiritual life. Seek the comfort of a supportive community, so that you might be refreshed with a new perspective to help you in your relationship with your Higher Power. Shut the door to guilt about how you're handling the situation. Try different forms of prayer that might speak to you more fully at this time. Know that whoever you are right now is the person you were created to be. Embrace and appreciate that self.

"When there is no enemy within, the enemies outside cannot hurt you."

African Proverb

CHAPTER NINE

Overtaxed and Overtired and You Can't Find the Light Switch

"Insanity is often the logic of an accurate mind overtaxed."

Oliver Wendell Holmes

There are days, and then there are days—days when everything seems to go pretty well, and days when nothing you do and nothing in the world around you is operating soundly. When depression is in the picture, you tend to have a lot more days of the latter than of the former. Depression takes a lot out of a person, whether that person is the one with the illness or the caregiver in the situation. What do you do when nothing is working, the darkness is closing in on you, and you can't find the light switch?

What Happens When Nothing Works?

We all have bad days. But when a person with depression is in your life, sometimes having a bad day can spell disaster.

Kelly's latest bad day started when her alarm didn't come on and she overslept. She had to hurry if she was going to make that important meeting first thing in the morning. Jake, her live-in partner, had been struggling with depression for more than five years. Last night, he had kept Kelly up late, talking about how terrible he felt and how he didn't know what to do next. Listening and finally getting him to agree to see the doctor earlier than scheduled had taken until two in the morning. Quickly kissing him, she wished him good luck with his doctor's visit and rushed out the door with their daughter, Angela, who was complaining because she didn't have enough time for breakfast. When they got into the car it wouldn't start, but with the usual coaxing the engine finally roared to life. When she dropped Angela off at school, her daughter's parting words were that Kelly had forgotten the cupcakes she'd promised to make for her class, which was supposed to celebrate Angela's birthday that day.

During the important meeting, Kelly had to keep apologizing about forgetting various items needed during the presentation. When the meeting finally ended, she returned to her desk to find five voice messages—one from her daughter's teacher about the cupcakes, and four from Jake, each longer and more mournful than the one before. After a day from hell at work, Kelly picked up Angela only to find her in tears because she hadn't been able to celebrate her birthday with her classmates. Kelly tried to make it up to her by taking her to a fast-food place, but Angela threw a tantrum when they didn't have the toy she wanted with her meal.

When Kelly and Angela got home, it was to find Jake in the bathroom with his pills spread out all around him, babbling to himself as to whether or not he should take them all. Exhausted and overwhelmed, Angela moved into a trancelike state, scooping up handfuls of pills and stuffing them back into whatever bottles were handy. Things continued to get worse. Jake refused to leave the bathroom, Angela threw up her fast-food meal, and Kelly realized she had left important papers at work. When she fell into bed at midnight next to Jake, she let the tears flow. Tomorrow promised to be just as bad.

Fending Off the Dark

We all have bad days, but living with a depressed loved one somehow makes those bad days even worse. Disaster is inevitable if we fail to take time for ourselves, if we don't ask for help in the day-to-day chores of life, if we think we can operate as we did before depression came into our home. We can't juggle everything on our own, and to tell ourselves we can is inviting trouble.

Avoiding the pitfalls requires planning and courage. Determine what absolutely needs to be done each day. Cut out as many items as you must. If you are not used to making yourself a schedule, now is the time to learn how. Write down everything, or make heavy use of whatever electronic calendar you have access to. When you are dealing with depression in the house, your mind has so much on it that it needs extra help keeping everything straight. Write down that those cupcakes are needed at school and on what date. Write down appointments and things you want to remember and then get in the habit of checking that calendar, each day looking at least two days ahead so you can be prepared. Send yourself emails, call your landline and cell phone, and leave yourself voice mails. Look at your calendar and your reminders as your lifelines. They will help to keep you sane during these seemingly insane times.

Meditation

"Stay centered, do not overstretch. Extend from your center, return to your center."

The Buddha

In our society we are often called to go above and beyond, stretching ourselves more than we should. As a result we find ourselves frazzled and unhappy, tense and irritable. When a depressed loved one is in the picture, these feelings are magnified.

Like muscles stretched beyond their capacity, when we are stretched beyond what we can and should do, we become unable to do our job. At those times we need to heal those mental muscles. We need to retreat into the center of our being and find calm. Once we find that calm, we are able to reach out again. Always, though, we must return to our center to restore the peace and calm that will enable our muscles to stretch as much as needed without damage.

Great Trainer, help me to realize the
importance of keeping my center strong.

Secondly, learn how the word "no" is said and practice it in front of a mirror if you need to. Saying no to some things is perhaps the healthiest thing you can do for yourself. When depression comes into the household we want to maintain a semblance of normalcy, and for far too many of us that normalcy involves saying yes to too many things. When we learn to say no we learn how to value our time and, therefore, ourselves. We can let someone else chair that important meeting. We can say no to helping on a field trip if it will cause too many complications for the family. We can say no to shopping for the neighbor, especially when getting our own shopping done can be overwhelming.

Don't be afraid to lower your standards for a while when you have this much stress in your life. Forego homemade birthday treats for something premade from the bakery. Learn to live with a dirty car if you're in too much of a time crunch to wash it. Give yourself permission to vacuum every other week, and turn a blind eye to the crumbs on the carpet in the meantime. You can always go back to your regular principles when times are better. Reducing the pressure you put on yourself can go a long way toward reducing your stress level.

Rest is another nonnegotiable. A depressed person can go on and on about his or her condition, going over the same territory time and time again. But you can only take so many conversations about depression, especially if they tend to crop up late in the evening. Learn to say no even in this arena. Don't let conversations start when bedtime rolls around. Emphasize to your loved one that good sleep helps you take better care of him or her and so the conversation will have to wait until you're up to it. Even if the request for a heart-to-heart comes during the day, you can say no if you simply don't have the emotional energy for it. Unless the person is indicating the possibility of suicide, let him or her know that what he or she has to say needs to wait for another time.

When children are involved, we must be honest with them about how off-kilter things are in the household. Don't hide it; you'll only make matters worse. Kids pick up on it pretty quickly when things aren't right. Letting them know the truth about what's happening helps them feel safe and stop worrying that they're to blame. Choose your words carefully, though, always remembering that they're children, not confidants. Talk to them in terms they can understand and go back to the topic as often as is necessary. Reassure them that though times are difficult due to depression, it will get better, and in the meantime you all must do the best you can.

Don't try to make things better by giving in to fast-food treats or other bribes, or by foregoing customary discipline for bad behavior. Kids need normalcy, routine, and boundaries. Enforcing regular bedtimes keeps everyone well rested and better able to deal with what's happening. Expecting chores to be done reminds kids that there's still order in the world and that they can contribute to keeping things going.

If it is your child who is the depressed person, it will be even more important to abide by these guidelines. Let him or her know you care, maintain boundaries, and expect responsible actions. Help your depressed child feel like a part of normal life.

Finally, make sure that you are taking time for your own self-care. Little things like a walk during the middle of the day, a bubble bath at day's end, coffee perked and ready when the day begins help you to take care of yourself during this time when depression is in your household. You'll find yourself less stressed and perhaps even happy.

Reflections

- *How do I feel when everything is going wrong?*

- *What aspects of a terrible day do I bring on myself?*

- *How can I love my depressed loved one through a bad day?*

Out-of-the-Ordinary Challenges

Depression is a major challenge all by itself. But clinical depression is not always the only diagnosis made. Other conditions often accompany it, and these tagalongs can create even more trouble.

Deb had been watching helplessly for some time as her husband, Scott, slid into depression. It began with the loss of his job after months of being in a probationary period with his boss; his concentration had slipped and he'd made major mistakes. Once he was finally fired, the melancholy moods, irritability, and sleepless nights had clued her in to the presence of depression. Deb had helped Scott find a therapist, monitored his antidepressant medications, and encouraged him to exercise. Things had improved a bit, but recently it seemed like new problems were cropping up at every turn.

Three months ago, after the depression symptoms had started to recede, Deb noticed that Scott's attention span had taken a nosedive. He fidgeted and complained any time he had to wait for anything. When faced with choices, even something as simple as what to put on his dinner plate, he became so frustrated and upset that he had to sit down for a while. As an elementary school teacher, Deb recognized several signs of attention deficit disorder. She convinced Scott to look into this possibility with their doctor, and a positive diagnosis came fairly quickly. Looking back, they both realized Scott's concentration and attention issues had been a problem for as long as they could remember. Apparently it was Scott's ability to navigate the difficulties that had changed. He began taking medication for ADD in addition to his antidepressants, and he and Deb both noticed an immediate improvement in his ability to concentrate and to handle choices that were in front of him.

But then, three times in two weeks, Scott was overtaken by spells of racing pulse, shaking, and obsessive thoughts that sent him into a state of terror. These episodes struck out of nowhere, and frightened both of them. Another trip to the doctor helped them discover that the ADD medications appeared to be triggering panic attacks. Scott tried a different prescription for the attention problem, but soon the panic attacks returned. Deb and Scott were faced with living either with the struggles of attention deficit disorder or with horrifying panic attacks. They chose to live with ADD, looking into behavioral changes Scott could make in order to manage the symptoms.

Through all these diagnoses, doctor visits, and scary episodes, Deb had stood alongside Scott. She was concerned for his health and happiness and longed for healing and a return to normal life. But the constant vigilance required, the assistance he needed in keeping track of medications and their consequences, the juggling of so many appointments—all the while keeping up with a full-time teaching job—were taking their toll on Deb. She found herself crying in the car every day on the way home from school. She snapped at Scott when he dithered over every tiny decision. She was having trouble sleeping, and her students' papers piled up as her energy level dropped and she stopped grading them each and every night, as had been her habit. Deb was nearing the end of her rope.

Other conditions, both physical and mental, can complicate depression. They may have been present all along, possibly contributing to the depression, or they may be by-products that show up after depression has appeared. Such complicating conditions can take the symptoms of depression out of the ordinary and create a picture that is difficult to read.

When the diagnoses start piling up, all of the coping skills we need as caregivers—PACT, self-care, awareness of the contagious aspect of depression—are even more essential. Whereas one issue can throw us off and make life difficult, multiple issues can send us into absolute chaos. Without lifelines such as community, a Higher Power, and attention to our own health, there's no way we can make it out of the darkness.

The presence of addiction, which frequently accompanies depression, creates more serious consequences. For instance, with the addition of alcohol or other recreational drugs, the medication for depression can be rendered either useless or too powerful. The mixture of drugs and alcohol might increase feelings of paranoia or of panic, or it might give the depression itself more power; when the drug wears off, the depression deepens.

If addiction rears its ugly head, extra help is needed. Encourage the depressed person to investigate and attend an appropriate twelve-step recovery program. Whether or not he or she does so, consider attending the appropriate twelve-step program (usually Al-Anon or Nar-Anon) for family members of addicts/alcoholics as a matter of self-care. As long as the addiction to alcohol or drugs is present, the depression cannot be addressed. Talk to the patient's psychologist or therapist about what should be done. Above all, watch for addiction and signs of depression in yourself. Whatever the manifestation of addiction, whether to food, alcohol, sex, or something else, addiction will never make a bad situation better.

Try This

Sometimes we forget just how hard it is to carry around extra resentment or addiction or anger. Take a couple of shopping bags and fill them with books or toys or whatever you have around the house. Now, for at least ten minutes, carry them around and try to do some type of cleaning project or work. Consider how it feels to be saddled with this extra unneeded material. Reflect on how the extra physical burden you experienced was like the extra resentment, anger, or addiction with which you were dealing.

Dealing with Zapped Energy, Enthusiasm, and Stamina

There's no way around it: living with depression in the household saps a person of energy, enthusiasm, and stamina. Not just the depressed person, but the whole household is affected. You find you don't feel like doing anything—going to the movies, reading a book, going to a friend's house. Eight hours of sleep just aren't enough, and sometimes you catch yourself feeling envious of the depressed person in your life, who can sleep ten, twelve, or sixteen hours. When you catch yourself doing that, it is time to take stock and change.

Enthusiasm comes from the Greek *en* and *theos,* meaning inspired by God. If your enthusiasm is lacking, maybe it's time you checked in with your Higher Power. When we try to do everything ourselves, when we look only to ourselves for the answers, we get nowhere. But when we let others help and look to our Higher Power for answers, we are able to move. Take a few moments, even if it is only two minutes, to be with your Higher Power. Open your heart and imagine God filling it with everything you need to strengthen you for that day. Let one of these strengths fill your being. Close your time with hugging yourself and imagine it is your Higher Power holding you in God's loving arms.

If you find your stamina lacking, turn to your support community. Maybe Ed has the staying power, Ellen is a great listener, Jane has resilience, Casey has energy, and Darla has strength. You can build up your stamina by letting that community of support do what they do best. Ed can stay with your depressed loved one when you need to get away. Ellen can listen when your loved one just has to talk and you can't bear to hear it anymore. Jane's resilience keeps you directed, giving you the strength to face one more day. Casey's energy proves to be contagious whenever you ask him over to help with something. When stuff is too much for you, Darla has the strength to listen and get you back on track. The community is full of stamina, those threads of energy that can see us through anything, if we only are willing to tap it.

Turning on That Light Switch

On days when it seems we can't take it any longer, those are the times when we need to stop and take advantage of the gifts around us. Turn to your Higher Power, bring in that community, affirm the worth of your time and energy by saying no, and tell yourself the truth: you need others if you are to do this, if you are to continue dancing toward health for you and your loved one.

CHAPTER TEN

Keeping Special Days in the Light

"We're fools whether we dance or not, so we might as well dance."

Japanese Proverb

Negativity is a hallmark of depression. The pessimism of a depressed person can taint all aspects of daily life, sapping us of joy and energy. It's hard to smile or have fun when someone close to us is frowning or lashing out in irritation. When we try to ignore the waves of negativity coming at us, when we try to dance in spite of the darkness, we can end up feeling guilty for leaving him or her behind, or our attempts to remain positive fall flat, overwhelmed by the effects of depression.

Holidays or special days such as birthdays and anniversaries can plunge a depressed person into an even deeper depression. Some have noted that just before or on the special day, the depressed individual will experience a crisis that makes it difficult or impossible for a celebration to occur. In extreme cases, the depressed person will deliberately plan something that can keep the focus on him or her. Depression has a tendency to make the sufferer intensely inwardly focused, unable to care or even notice that others might wish to celebrate and enjoy special times.

This type of behavior can have several effects. The nondepressed persons might question whether they are entitled to feel good when someone they love is feeling so bad. They may wonder why they are not appreciated, why they can't have the perfect holiday like everyone else around them seems to have. They might attempt to celebrate in spite of the negative emotions, but perceive the celebration as spoiled by the feeling of walking on eggshells, trying to placate the depressed person. How, then, can we continue to celebrate holidays, birthdays, and other special days without putting more strain on an already strained relationship?

Celebrating Together

It was New Year's Eve. The family was scheduled to go to a friend's house to celebrate the holiday with games and goodies. Everything was set. The kids were excited at the idea of seeing their friends. The mom, Sherry, was looking forward to a relaxing and fun evening. But then the father, Stan, declared that they wouldn't be going. His depression, he said, made it too hard for him to be with so many people.

Sherry thought about the consequences for her, for the children, and for her husband, and came to a decision. She would take the children to the party and Stan could stay at home where he wanted to be. Trying carefully to not let anger enter into her tone, she stated to her husband that she and the kids were going to the party even if he didn't want to go. He could stay at home and watch the ball drop on television and they would be home when the party was winding down.

Stan stayed at home. When the rest of the family returned they told him about their evening and asked him about what he had watched on TV. This family successfully navigated the celebration of the holiday without leaving anyone out. Stan did what he wanted and was able to share it with his family on their return and to hear their stories as well. Although the interest on his part might not have been the greatest, he was at least able to be included in the holiday in some small way. Sherry and the kids enjoyed themselves and could return to the situation at home with a more positive and supportive attitude. Their happiness was tempered because

Stan couldn't join them, but the celebration had taken place even though he hadn't been there.

Holidays, for any family, are times of negotiations. For a family living with a depressed person, considering creative options can be an important tool for remaining healthy and happy. The holiday may not look the way it has in the past, but with care, it can still be a satisfying time for all.

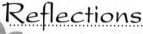

Reflections

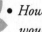

- *How can I talk with the depressed person to find out what would be his or her preference during a holiday time?*

- *How can we look at a holiday differently and still help everyone to celebrate in a way that is good for them?*

Reducing the Stress of Celebratory Times

It's a fact that times of celebration and joy can bring along their share of stress. In our efforts to make a day special, we tend to go overboard, trying to fit in more than we can comfortably pull off. A day of celebration at Christmas turns into a month of trying to create the perfect experience: baked treats, parties, perfect gifts, shining decorations. A child's birthday turns into a circus of too many guests, too many presents, and overly elaborate and expensive activities. If we're not mindful of our own limitations, by the time the special day is over we're so tired from the production we've created that we have little energy left to enjoy ourselves.

This state of affairs is one we can't afford when we're dealing with depression. Our time and energy are already sapped in dealing with the depressed person's illness; our checkbooks may already be stretched as we try to cover the costs of treatment. It's time to downsize our celebrations.

First, we have to take a fresh look at what makes a particular day special. What can we absolutely not leave out if we want it to be a true celebration? What is extra "fat" that can be trimmed without depriving us of a happy time? Sticking to only the necessities that we can comfortably manage is a must.

Try This

Before a holiday, make a "holiday tip sheet." If there are children in the household, have them decorate the page. Each member of the family, sometime in the days before the holiday, writes or draws what they would like to do to make the holiday special and happy. Just before the holiday, the family can consider the ideas on the tip sheet, each member choosing one thing to do. Those individual items are the only things that happen on the holiday. Anything else is extra. Negotiating skills and creativity may be required to ensure that each item is possible. But in the end everyone gets something they want and no one—the depressed person included—is excluded.

Downsizing our celebration requires us to reassess our priorities. In the end, what's more important—that the house looks like something out of a magazine, or that everyone involved comes away with a happy memory? When the celebration is over, how do we want each person to feel—exhausted from the strain of entertaining, or peaceful in knowing that happy memories were made? Getting down to the essence of why we're celebrating can help us create a time that allows dancing in spite of depression.

Preparation and Practice

When a special time is coming up, thinking ahead can help you avoid difficulties down the road. Practice, before a mirror if necessary, talking about the approaching holiday and how it might affect each person. Imagine the responses, and imagine not only listening to those responses but also reacting to them in a positive way for everyone concerned. Whether or not children are involved, consider what the adults in the relationship need to do to prepare for the holiday. Decide together what each of you wants to do for the holiday. What needs to be done to make this possible?

Sometimes it is difficult to talk to a depressed person. He or she may have great challenges expressing their feelings, or their words may be consistently negative. Running through a conversation in your mind ahead of time will help you as you have the actual conversation. A good conversation with the depressed person can lead to a good celebration for all concerned.

Dealing with Sabotage

Whether they intend to or not, depressed people can put the kibosh on a celebration before it even gets going. It may be that they're overwhelmed by the prospect of extra work and extra people in the house, causing them to plunge into an emotional state that renders them incapable of celebration. Or it may be that they're so mired in the negativity that accompanies depression that they can't bear to see others feeling happy. Whatever is behind it, the actions and moods of a depressed person can seem like sabotage.

From the time she was little, Alice loved birthdays. She thought it was a day to celebrate the person and, in a way, thank them for being in the lives of others. Her partner in their early years together agreed that birthdays were special, but over the past two years Jonathan had been battling depression and had become inwardly focused, so much so that he would joke feebly that it was "all about me." Alice decided that despite Jonathan's depression, she would still celebrate her own approaching birthday by inviting friends over and having a small party.

On the day of the party, with everything ready and only a few hours to the arrival of guests, Jonathan announced that he felt absolutely horrible. The depression, he said, had gotten so much worse, he couldn't imagine coming out of it. Alice listened, seeing Jonathan disintegrate before her eyes, crying and bemoaning how horrible he felt. There was nothing to do but to cancel the party. Another birthday uncelebrated. Alice reflected later that night that it had also occurred on their anniversary, her birthday the previous year, and the day she found out her watercolor was chosen as the best in a local art show. Depression was killing all of Alice's life celebrations.

We deserve to celebrate the good times in life. If your depressed partner is unable to do so, speak up ahead of time to let them know you understand, but that it is important to you to celebrate these milestones in your life. Then, go ahead and celebrate. It is one of the ways you can renew your own spirit so you can continue to help your loved one heal.

Meditation

"Success is measured not so much by the position that one has reached in life as by the obstacles which one has overcome while trying to succeed."

Booker T. Washington

Picture yourself biking through a landscape marked by hills and valleys, on a beautiful spring day. Parts of the ride are arduous, even painful, as your leg muscles pump their hardest to reach the peak of the next hill. You're almost ready to give up when you reach the top of the hill. From this height, you're able to see more hills and a patchwork of colors in the foliage below. You feel a soft and cooling breeze on your cheek. You hear the joyful song of wild birds. It was worth the effort, just to get to this place.

Now it's time to head down to the next valley. This is an easy ride at first, as no effort is needed to coast downward. But before you know it you pick up more speed than you like. You're careening down the hill, frightened that any little bump in the road will send you tumbling to the bottom. Finally you make your way to the lowest point, where the lovely sights and sounds of the hilltop have disappeared. You'll have to make another difficult climb up the next hill to experience that beauty again—but the memory of the beauty you enjoyed at the top gives you the energy to do just that.

This imaginary ride is much like what we experience in life. Ordinary days, months, and years are punctuated by exhilarating views as we celebrate joyous times with those we love. Much of our time is spent in getting to a place where we can celebrate. But some of our time is also spent in fear and concern as the low places, such as caring for a depressed person, loom ahead. We need to drink in the experience of joy on the hilltops to keep us going when we hit the valleys.

Higher Power, allow me to be fully present in
times of joy, that I may be able to use this joy
to get me through the low points of life.

Celebrating with or without Your Partner

Close friends invited Annie and Jason over for an end-of-summer dessert and pool party. It had been a long, tough week of errands, evening meetings, and puzzling over how to cover the mortgage. An evening of relaxation by the pool with people who had stuck with them through good and bad was exactly what Jason needed, especially since Annie seemed to be making little progress with her treatment for depression.

The invitation was for 7:00 p.m., and by 6:45 Jason was ready to head out. But as he reached for his keys, he discovered that Annie hadn't put on her swimsuit; in fact, she hadn't even risen from her place on the couch. She seemed to be in no hurry to get changed and go along. The ensuing conversation sounded something like this:

"It's 6:45. Time to go. Aren't you coming? I thought you wanted to come."

"I do."

Silence.

"Well, I don't want to be late. Let's go."

(Deep sigh.) "Okay." (No movement.)

"Are you coming or not?"

More silence.

Jason had a decision to make. It wasn't the first time this had happened— Annie, sometimes paralyzed by the depression that had been with her for months, made them late to events that were important to them. This time, Jason made a choice that he hadn't tried in the past. Jason went on to the pool party, leaving Annie behind to follow on her own timetable. He tried his best to make his decision clear in a nonjudgmental way, telling her he hoped she'd be along soon, and he'd let everyone know she'd come as soon as she could. He just needed to be part of this celebration with friends, whether she came along or not.

Depressed people seem to have no sense of time. They're chronically late for appointments. A trip to the corner store for two or three items can turn into a two-hour absence. A chore that would take a well person twenty minutes might take a depressed person an entire day. Confusion and muddled thinking prevent them from operating on the same schedule as those who are not depressed. A lot of friction can result as we try to live with this.

Chances are, if this situation sounds familiar to you, there's a conversation you need to have with the depressed person sometime soon, when you *aren't* trying to get to an event that both of you would normally enjoy. That conversation could center around the possibility of choosing to go to the event on your own time and allowing your partner to arrive whenever he or she is ready, or it could involve choosing to do activities at a time of day that is more comfortable for the depressed person. For example, if she has more difficulty in the morning, you might plan activities for the afternoon and evening hours as much as possible.

Once you've considered these possibilities in the cool of an unrushed moment, create in your mind a proposal you might present to your partner. A conversation ahead of time might forestall feelings of frustration next time you plan to go out.

Reflections

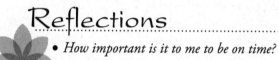

- *How important is it to me to be on time?*

- *How do I feel about attending social events without my spouse?*

- *How might we make going out easier for both of us?*

Celebrating Your Relationship

It was their two-year anniversary, and Sharon had hoped something might change that would allow them to enjoy the special day together. Instead, the day began with Theresa staying in bed until almost noon, on the heels of her promise that she would get up early that day and look at the classifieds in the paper. Then she didn't eat anything, saying she wasn't hungry. Next came complaints about how dirty the house was. Sharon left to run errands, a tactic she often used to avoid arguments with her partner, returning to find Theresa sleeping in front of the television. When Sharon woke her, she yelled at Sharon for waking her from a sound sleep, and returned to complaining about the house. She didn't eat any dinner even though Sharon fixed her favorite meal, with candles and flowers on the table, which she'd bought to mark what was supposed to be a special day. Theresa was in bed again well before nine p.m. Why do I stay with her? Sharon asked herself. She hasn't worked in months; she yells at me all the time. Obviously this milestone in our relationship doesn't mean much to her. Everything was all about Theresa, and Sharon was sick and tired of it all.

Depressed people can be hard to love. The illness seems to erase the qualities we had originally enjoyed and appreciated in them, replacing them with traits that are unattractive at best. We find ourselves wondering, as Sharon did, how we can celebrate the relationship together when the person we originally committed to appears to have disappeared.

In this confusing and painful time, it can help to take a giant step backward and look at the situation and the relationship from a distance. Go for a walk, go out to a movie, or even take a weekend trip alone to do something pleasurable. Simply getting time away from him or her can allow us to return with a renewed ability to handle the difficulties of depression. While you're having some time away, make a conscious effort to remember what was previously good and positive about this person and about your relationship.

Seek out people you can talk to about how hard things are right now. Unloading the frustration and hurt to a trusted third party can be a lifeline. At this time, when your relationship looks so very different than it did during good times, you need to create some distance that can let in light and energy, allowing you to keep dancing together through the darkness.

Reflections

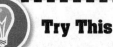

- *Think back. What was it that initially attracted you to your partner?*

- *What were at least three of the qualities that you appreciated about him or her?*

- *What qualities are you missing most now?*

- *What positive qualities does your partner still exhibit toward you or others?*

Try This

Sit down and write out your partner's full name. Now, taking each individual letter, write a quality that you have seen, see now, or might see in the future from your partner. Work as hard as you can to use all of the letters in your partner's name. When you are done—whether or not you have a full list—take some time to reflect on the qualities. Recall times when you were especially aware of those qualities in your partner. Take time to remember that these qualities have not gone away. Depression is hiding them.

Rely on PACT at this time. When you are in communication with your Higher Power and your community of support, it is difficult to plunge into the depths because so many hands are holding you up. Time taken regularly with your Higher Power can remind you of the meaning and purpose in life; life is more than the negativity of depression. A phone call or lunch with a trusted friend will help to keep you afloat when it seems like an important person in your life is plunging deeper into the abyss. Share with someone what is going on regarding the upcoming holiday or special day. Get ideas about what can be done to make the holiday enjoyable for all of you, from someone who's not affected by the depression. Allow those outside the circle of depression to celebrate with you in a healthy way.

Remember your PACT with your Higher Power:

Prayer

Affirmation

Community

Truth

Above all, don't allow depression to keep you from participating in the joyful dance of life.

Dealing with the Dark Side

> "Bad company is like a nail driven into a post, which, after the first
> and second blow, may be drawn out with little difficulty; but being
> once driven up to the head, the pincers cannot take hold to draw it
> out, but which can only be done by the destruction of the wood."

Saint Aurelius Augustine

We all want those we love to get better. We want to see life for them
return to being full and trouble-free. When depression is part of day-
to-day life, returning to a fulfilling life is not easy. Depression may eat away
at the very fabric of your relationship with your loved one. It can take away
the good feelings you had and replace them with negative ones. Depression
sometimes takes away any hope that our loved one will get better and leaves
us with the feeling that somehow or other, we have failed. The sad fact
is that sometimes, despite our best efforts to use medication and therapy
and support, depression refuses to lift. The roller-coaster ride may take an
emotional toll on the caregiver, causing the relationship to break, or our
loved one may become consumed with addictions that complicate care
as well as complicating the relationship. It's hard to deal with all of these
possibilities and still keep a relationship alive and vibrant. Sometimes it just
can't work.

Divorce

The end of a relationship is rarely a sought-after choice. Nevertheless, it is a choice that sometimes has to be made in a relationship where depression plays a major part.

Jan and Archie had been married for twenty-seven years. They shared many interests and enjoyed each other's company—that is, when the depression wasn't present. Jan had struggled with depression for many years. She had tried many medication combinations and had gone through hours of therapy. But what she could not or would not accept was the reality of being on medication permanently, if she was to experience anything like a healthy life. Instead, whenever she was feeling good, she gradually—at first unbeknownst to her husband or her doctor—stopped taking the medication. Each time she would slip into a depression of greater depth than the last. Each time she would let out her frustration in varying expressions of anger, each a more violent expression than the last episode.

Despite Archie's pleas, Jan refused to stay on the medicine, reasoning that she was better and didn't need it. However, when Jan took a knife to Archie during an especially difficult time, Archie knew he couldn't keep on like this. As tough at it was, he decided on separation, figuring that it would be the jolt needed to spur Jan into listening to her doctors' advice. Unfortunately, things only got worse. Not only did Jan stop taking her medicine, but she also turned to alcohol to numb her feelings about the loss of Archie. Finally Archie filed for divorce, realizing he could no longer be of help to her. He knew too that although he would always love her, he could not continue to live with her. As the days went by he liked her less and less. She had become, for him, a "crazymaker."

Crazymakers tear at us with negativity, keeping us from being ourselves. Sometimes people with depression are crazymakers in the lives of those who are close to them. Even in times of reason, they do not accept that changes must be made for the sake of the other person. Often they feel everything is "all about them" and they fail to even consider the needs and concerns of others. They may be emotionally unable to look outside themselves, or they may consciously think their own pain is too great to take others into account. This way of thinking and operating contributes to the breakdown of a relationship.

The crazymakers in relationships already burdened with depression are not the only ones who may struggle with addiction, however. In an effort to escape the pain of depression, people struggling with the illness have a disproportionately high tendency to turn to alcohol, other drugs, or sexual addictions to "self-medicate." Obviously, addictions throw an already off-balance relationship even more off-kilter.

In some cases, the loved one cannot do anything about the fact that depression does not dissipate. He or she does everything the doctors recommend. If therapy is suggested, he or she dutifully participates. He or she accepts the love and support of family and friends and still doesn't get better. Sometimes he or she even feels worse. Eventually a couple struggling with one partner's depression might mutually agree that divorce is the only option. A fresh start might be something both of them need.

Divorce, whether mutually agreed upon or a decision the caregiver must make on his or her own, is sometimes the outcome of depression. We all like to think that our marriages or long-term relationships will survive, but sometimes, for the sake of safety or for emotional health and growth, divorce or separation is the only choice. It is never easy to end a committed relationship, but when arguments ramp up and any children are put in danger or when addiction surfaces, the factors pointing toward divorce as a solution become difficult to ignore. There are situations in which physical or emotional safety, health, or other factors make divorce inevitable. In other situations, when abuse, addiction, or other problems with severe consequences are not present, the option of a trial separation may be better.

Questions to Consider Before Divorce

These questions are just a few to consider if you are contemplating divorce:

- What are the most prevalent feelings you have now about your partner? What were your feelings earlier in the relationship?

- How has depression affected your consideration of divorce?

- What things have changed to move you toward divorce?

- What do you need to do (financially, emotionally, logistically) to be prepared for life after the divorce?

- What will you miss about your relationship after the divorce? How will you deal with this loss?

If divorce is, in the end, the best decision, try to end the relationship as amicably as possible. Due to the presence of depression, take extra care in the ending, so the depressed person is able to continue moving forward after you're gone. Make it clear to your loved one that you care about them, will always care about them, but for your own sanity and safety you need to move on. Do whatever you can to leave your loved one with a caring support network of people who will continue to help in whatever way they can. Make sure at least one other person knows the course of treatment and the present medications that are part of your loved one's life. If you are healthy enough mentally, make arrangements to see your loved one on a regular basis and, if children are present in the relationship, for them also to continue to see the loved one. Make an attempt to consult with the depressed person's therapist so that person can come up with a plan for handling life after you are gone. Consider finding a therapist for yourself to help you handle the roller coaster of emotion that you are likely to experience during this time.

However, we don't always live in a perfect world. It might be necessary to just leave the relationship, especially if circumstances are present that endanger emotional or physical health, growth, or even financial solvency. You've done all you can, and you must move on to preserve your own health and well-being. Again, seek out a good therapist or friend who will help you work through any feelings of anger or guilt. Remind yourself time and time again: sometimes it is just necessary to leave a situation for the good of all individuals involved.

Divorce does not have to be bitter and ugly. Whether we are able to do it amicably or we have to leave abruptly, we can do what we can to make it a positive move for all involved, despite the pain of the end of the relationship. Divorce is sometimes an opportunity for better health for all involved.

**"Was I deceiv'd, or did a sable cloud
Turn forth her silver lining on the night?"**

John Milton

Estrangement

Estrangement happens in many different ways. It can happen suddenly, with some emotional explosion that causes people to avoid each other. It can happen slowly, insidiously, with the fact that they have become estranged coming as a late-dawning surprise. With depression in the mix, it might take us even longer to recognize it, whether it comes quickly or slowly.

Stella had taken care of her mother, Edna, for more than two years, and she was exhausted. Whenever she attempted to take some time for herself, her mother invariably had a crisis. As much as she tried, Stella could not get her mother to realize there were other people around who could help her. So Stella, ever the dutiful daughter, continued to take care of her mom. She ran errands for Edna, and every time Stella returned, her mother would be particularly cruel with comments about her appearance, about what she had purchased, about her relationships. By the time Stella left her mother's house, she felt as if she had gone through a battle. When Edna had to go to the doctor, she embarrassed Stella, harping on her daughter's own health issues when the doctor came into the room. When Stella tried to talk with her about it, her mother refused to listen. Gradually, Stella came to dread having any interaction with her mother at all. She didn't need to be mentally abused, she felt, by a woman who could do a lot of these things herself but just didn't care to. More and more, Stella came to dislike her mother, finding excuses not to see her until finally she ended all contact with her. She arranged for a nurse, and when that brought brutal phone calls, she changed her number and even stopped calling to see how her mother was doing. Soon, it seemed as if her mother had already died— which she had, in Stella's mind.

Estrangement can happen even if we don't want it to. Our depressed loved one might be so difficult and so negative that it happens slowly as a result of our avoiding each other more and more. Or there might be an ugly scene that brings things to a head all at once. We one day realize we are worn out from being abused, and we simply put an end to contact. We have had enough, and we react as we feel we must, in self-preservation. Estrangement from loved ones isn't what we might wish, but it sometimes becomes the only option.

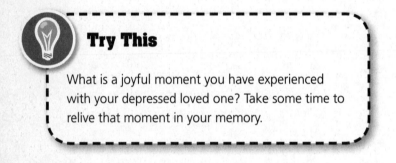

Try This

What is a joyful moment you have experienced with your depressed loved one? Take some time to relive that moment in your memory.

Sometimes there is nothing we can do to maintain a relationship and maintain our own emotional health, as well. There may be issues in the person's past about which we're unaware. We may or may not ever learn what causes a person to become so toxic that we can no longer be in relationship with them. However, we were not meant to be emotional (or actual) punching bags. If we're interested in finding a way to keep the relationship alive on some level, we have to deal with the situation with an eye toward permanent, positive changes.

It might help to remind yourself that you have, in effect, become the parent in the relationship. Coming to terms with this role and all that goes with it can help you look at the situation from a different perspective. Remind yourself that, at least during this time of depression, you are the responsible adult. It is up to you to create boundaries, to establish expectations, and to set the tone for what your relationship should look like. At the same time, as any good parent would do, you need to provide consequences for unacceptable behavior—any behavior that makes you feel abused, belittled, or unappreciated.

> **"A person isn't who they are during the last conversation you had with them—they're who they've been throughout your whole relationship."**
>
> Rainer Maria Rilke

First of all, if possible, talk with your loved one about the fact that you are feeling mistreated. It is an excellent idea to have a third party present to help facilitate the conversation. Spell out your concerns. Point out how these things are hurtful to you and that you don't want this to come between the two of you. Be clear about what you can and cannot do. Determine the amount of time you can reasonably devote to caring for the person. Explain that when you are spoken to disrespectfully, if you're not appreciated and treated with simple courtesy, or in the event of any other behavior that makes you miserable, you must, for the sake of your own well-being, distance yourself for a time, finding others who can step in and assist your loved one while you have time away.

If, after this conversation, you continue to find yourself feeling abused, make a point to talk to a trusted friend, both to unload and to get a new perspective and new ideas. As you go forward, go out of your way to deliberately recall your loved one's good qualities, remembering that this person is more than the ugly behavior that's been caused by depression. Follow through with the solutions you discuss and the consequences that must ensue. Creating healthy boundaries in this way might help you save the relationship.

In Times of Darkness

Sometimes people have so many hurts, have fallen into such particular ways of behaving and responding, that it makes a meaningful conversation extremely difficult, if not impossible. With certain persons, a letter spelling out what you see happening and how you're feeling is more effective than a verbal conversation. In writing, each individual can consider his or her responses and answer more thoughtfully.

But there are times when a relationship simply cannot be saved. Then, as they say in Westerns, "it's time to get out of Dodge." When you've done all you can but come to realize that nothing you say or do will make any difference, you need to salvage what you can of the relationship. In this case, you will have to draw back completely and turn over the care of the person to other individuals who are able to handle it. This is an extremely difficult course of action, raising a great many guilt feelings that can cause you to backtrack on the promises you made to care for yourself. Make every attempt to say calmly to the person, "I love you, and I cannot allow you to treat me this way any longer. In fact, I love you enough to not let you damage our relationship any further." It's very difficult to do, but sometimes it's the only option. Write it out beforehand, if necessary. Practice saying it into a mirror or to someone you can trust, to make it easier to say to the person in question.

The decision to remove yourself from a relationship can be extremely wearing. Once you've distanced yourself, your loved one might not take care of him- or herself. He or she might be hard on the people coming in to help. You might see your loved one doing things that hurt you even at a distance; it can be difficult not to step in and step back into the dance that chipped away at self esteem, love, and happiness. You have to create a new dance, one that keeps your partner at a distance instead of close to you. If you do this for your own health and well-being, the healing that results may ease the estrangement. Even if it doesn't, the new dance helps us to be better, healthier human beings, ready to love and reach out, knowing that we have done all we could for the people we love.

Estrangement doesn't have to last a lifetime or turn to enmity, as it did for the legendary Hatfields and McCoys. You can reconnect once health returns; you can build that relationship back up. It will take time and talk and understanding, but it can be done. Once healing has occurred, make an effort to look at your loved ones with fresh eyes, seeing them in a new light, and listen—really listen—to what they are saying. Bit by bit, you can rebuild the relationship, always looking to your Higher Power for guidance.

Reflections

- *What is the most prominent feeling for you during this dark period?*

- *In what areas of your life do you feel estranged?*

- *What are you willing to do for a healthier relationship?*

- *If there is an estrangement, what are you doing to handle it?*

Suicide

Through the ages, suicide has been a taboo subject, often misunderstood and always frightening. Churches had prohibitions against burying in sacred ground the bodies of people who had committed suicide. Families of those who committed suicide were shunned socially. People whispered behind backs: "She committed suicide. Isn't that terrible? Why didn't anyone do anything?" People would speculate as to what would cause a person to take his or her own life. There was the feeling that the shame and horror might be contagious.

Some of these attitudes have changed, but not all. Suicide still carries the stigma of being the ultimate evil, something unthinkable to the average person. But the reality is that suicide sadly is sometimes the outcome of depression, much the same as death is sometimes the outcome of cancer or some other disease. It's not contagious, it doesn't have to be hidden, and people are not terrible if they succumb. At the same time, not all depressed individuals commit suicide, and not all suicides are a result of depression. Sometimes a catastrophic event or serious illness might cause an individual to turn to suicide. We as caregivers do our best to prevent it, but we need to remember we are not all-powerful or all-controlling.

For many people who are depressed, suicide is not about wanting to die; rather, it is about wanting the pain to stop. It is a call for freedom from the hurt and the hopelessness. It is a desire for release from the mental torment that often overtakes a depressed individual. In short, the person doesn't want to die. They want to live, but how to do so is lost in the fog of depression.

Meditation

"Far away, there in the sunshine are my highest aspirations. I may not reach them, but I can look up and see their beauty, believe in them, and try to follow where they lead."

Louisa May Alcott

One of the things that occurs with depression is the growth of feelings of hopelessness and helplessness. Sometimes the despair is so great that thoughts of ending one's life are ever-present. When someone we love has these thoughts, we feel helpless. We question what we could do to make it better. We want our loved one to see that there is much to live for, much to do in life. In these moments of sheer darkness, we have to remember that even if it is far, far away, there is sunshine, there is hope. Sadly, the person we love can't always reach the sunshine, cannot see the beauty in and even ends the relationship we have with them, or, at the worst, ends life itself. We have to remember at those times that depression is an illness, and as with any illness sometimes it takes a long time for people to get better. Sometimes they do not get better. Divorce or estrangement, and sometimes suicide, result. Our Higher Power asks us to remember that there is always beauty in life. No matter the outcome of the illness, that person still had many good, beautiful moments in life. No matter the darkness, we can celebrate joy and beauty and look to the sunshine.

*Loving Supporter, help me in my darkest
time to remember that there is sunshine
waiting for me and those I love.*

Prevention

In any circumstance, suicide or talk of suicide is serious business. We, the authors, are not doctors, and we certainly don't have all the answers. If you judge that there is the possibility of suicide, contact the depressed person's doctor or therapist, being aware that they may not be able to breach their patient's confidentiality unless such discussions have been previously agreed upon by all parties. There are general guidelines caregivers should keep in mind.

At times, depressed people may attempt to hide thoughts of suicide from their therapist or prescribing doctor. They feel unable to have the discussion; they fear the consequences, such as hospitalization. They may wish to keep the thought to themselves in order to allow it to remain an option. It's possible you need to be the one to contact a medical professional should you suspect that your loved one is not being honest about suicidal thoughts.

When addressing suicide prevention, note that different depressed people exhibit different symptoms or warning signs. If suicide is a concern for your loved one, familiarize yourself with the general symptoms. But look at the warning signs through the lens of your loved one's personality. Consider how he or she would likely express the warning signs according to his or her individual character.

Some of the ways a person planning suicide might express the intention could include:

- Complaints of being a bad person or comments about feeling terrible inside.

- Despondency over major loss that has happened in their life, such as divorce, breakup, family trauma, news of illness.

- Verbal comments such as "Nobody cares" or "I can't take it any longer."

- Moves to put affairs in order, whether that is a teenager giving a prized possession to a friend or an elderly individual reworking his or her will.

- Signs of hopelessness—"I just want this to end."

- Direct statements that point directly to the intent to kill themselves.

There are several things to consider as means of prevention if your loved one is showing suicidal tendencies:

Remember the "T" of PACT

One form of suicide prevention is present in the "T" of PACT. Tell the truth about the possibility of suicide. Don't be afraid to talk about it. Ask your loved one if he or she has thoughts of suicide. Research has shown that just because you talk about suicide doesn't mean that it is going to happen. Quite the opposite is true. Truth brings the thought out into the light so that it can be dealt with. Bring that truth to the forefront if your loved one has spoken of suicide. Ask them before you leave them alone, "Are you safe alone right now?" Keep the subject in the light.

Consider a Contract of Protection

The subject of suicide should never be taken lightly. Because it is a real possibility when depression is present, consider a contract of protection with each other. Such a contract allows each of you to feel there is something that is standing in the way of your loved one following through on a suicidal thought. Often called a "no-suicide contract," it is essentially an agreement in which your loved one promises not to hurt him- or herself. If the eventuality that suicide is imminent, the contract contains a previously agreed-upon contingency plan for possible prevention. Here is an example:

A Sample No-Suicide Contract (Contract of Protection)

I, _____, agree that I will not attempt to cause harm to myself.

If I am ever having thoughts of suicide, am feeling like I want to kill myself, and/or have the urge to cause harm to myself:

1. I will remind myself that _____ and _____ care deeply for me and do not want me to harm myself.

2. I will remind myself that I can never attempt to commit suicide.

3. I will call 911 immediately if I feel that I could hurt myself that day.

4. I will call the following phone numbers if I am feeling suicidal, but do not feel that I will cause harm to myself immediately.
   (List contact names and numbers.)

5. If I am feeling like I want to die and/or commit suicide and cannot reach the above persons, I will call 1-800-SUICIDE.

I know that _____ and _____ do not want me to hurt myself, and care about me very much.

Signed _____

This contract is by no means a fail-safe way to prevent suicide, but it does allow the subject to stay in the open, and it may serve as a deterrent long enough for help to be sought.

Know the Facts About Suicide

When we are well-informed about a subject, we feel better able to talk about it or to act on the information. Knowing the facts enables us to act in positive ways with our loved ones. We know when and where to go for help and what to say and what not to say. Being armed with this information can help in a crucial time.

- Always take a person who expresses suicidal thoughts seriously. Granted, he or she might only want attention, but you are not trained to know the difference. Assume it is a serious thought.

- Don't give advice. Just listen. Give support and encouragement and avoid the use of the word "should"; "shoulds" only encourage guilt. A person considering suicide is already filled with guilt.

- Suggest ways in which you can help. Ask if the person is willing to go to the doctor, and offer to go along for support. Talk about a plan for the coming days—whom he or she could call, how he or she might get through each day—and let them know you will be there for them.

- If you are concerned about suicide, seek professional help immediately. Don't think that your loved one will work it out for him- or herself.

If the threat of suicide is part of your life with your loved one, be aware of your own feelings. Find people, both professionals and trusted friends, to talk to about the situation. Remind yourself that the issue of suicide is part of the disease of depression. It is normal to feel anger at times and to have thoughts of having failed your loved one. Take into account the "C" in PACT and call the people in the community to help and support you and your loved one. Remember the "P" in PACT as well: keep in touch with your Higher Power, asking your Higher Power to give you the strength and insight to deal with this very difficult part of depression.

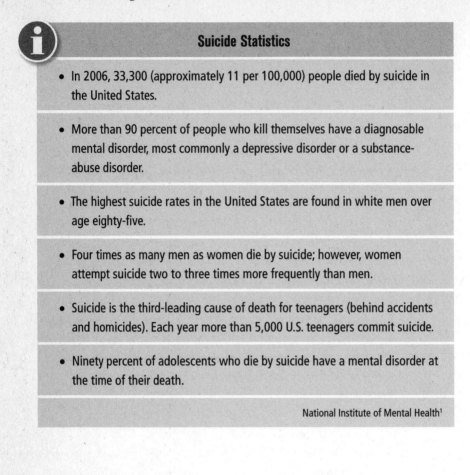

Suicide Statistics

- In 2006, 33,300 (approximately 11 per 100,000) people died by suicide in the United States.

- More than 90 percent of people who kill themselves have a diagnosable mental disorder, most commonly a depressive disorder or a substance-abuse disorder.

- The highest suicide rates in the United States are found in white men over age eighty-five.

- Four times as many men as women die by suicide; however, women attempt suicide two to three times more frequently than men.

- Suicide is the third-leading cause of death for teenagers (behind accidents and homicides). Each year more than 5,000 U.S. teenagers commit suicide.

- Ninety percent of adolescents who die by suicide have a mental disorder at the time of their death.

National Institute of Mental Health[1]

When the Worst Happens

When suicide becomes the fatal outcome of the disease of depression, it leaves overwhelming emotional turmoil in its wake. Moving on in life is very difficult indeed. Anger wells up. The sense of loss is great. Survivors are riddled with feelings of failure, wondering what they could have done differently. Life will never be the same after suicide, and a new "normal" must be found. The presence of a professionally trained person to help survivors deal with the aftermath of suicide is strongly recommended.

Try This

Make a list of things that make living worthwhile. Read it over as often as you need to in order to remember that life is indeed good, and loving people is the best part.

Remembering PACT at this time is especially helpful.

Pray to your Higher Power. Pour out your feelings, place yourself in the Higher Power's loving arms. Keeping in touch with your Higher Power will give you the strength each and every day to make a choice to let go of the guilt and the "could haves," "would haves," and "should haves."

Affirmation reminds you that you are a good person, that what happened to your loved one was a choice that he or she made. Affirmation will help you remember that you did what you could and that life is good and worth living.

Community is vital at a time of suicide. You need people around you to remind you of your worth, to remind you of everything you have done for your loved one, to give you the emotional support that will see you through this difficult time.

Truth will remind you that sometimes suicide is just the natural outcome of this wicked disease we call depression. Truth will also help you acknowledge the anger and hurt you feel because a loved one has done this to you. Truth will give you permission to say it is okay to be angry about what your loved one did.

Suicide is devastating to the loved ones who survive. Teaching ourselves to remember the funny moments, the warm moments with our loved one, the good times we had together, will help us heal. Everything was not terrible, everything was not dire, and when we remember that, we can see that life is good and that loving another is the best part no matter how badly it may end or how it may hurt right now.

CHAPTER ELEVEN NOTES

1. National Institute of Mental Health. 2007 [Online]. Available from http://www.nimh.nih.gov/health/publications/suicide-in-the-us-statistics-and-prevention/index.shtml (accessed 18 March 2011).

CHAPTER TWELVE

Recovering and Recognizing the Light

"To watch us dance is to hear our hearts speak."

Hopi Saying

W e've all experienced storms—the night filled with crashes of thunder and lightning, torrential rains, and violent winds. Then comes the morning sun peeking over the horizon, its strong rays slowly but surely covering the landscape. Little blades of grass twinkle with the last remnants of the rain, and the air is filled with the sound of birds twittering as they hop from branch to branch. The beauty of the aftermath of a storm is an experience to savor, to revel in with each tiny discovery as you let the warmth of the new day seep down into the depths of your being.

Recovery from depression is similar to coming out of a terrible storm into the light of new life and newness all around you. People who are depressed do get better. More than 80 percent of those people who seek treatment for depression do indeed recover. With the right medication and the right therapy, they can come to a stage of happiness they may never have felt before. For us caregivers, this time of recovery holds a number of surprises.

The Exhilaration of Wellness

Kim did a double-take as she lay in bed. The clock said seven a.m., a time when George was usually in bed beside her. Every morning for years she'd had to coax him awake and keep up a steady stream of dialogue as he dressed so that he would complete the task at hand and be ready to face the day. George had been battling depression for more than three years, and Kim had fallen into a routine that helped him to function, at least in a modified way. But this morning was different. He was taking a shower, and wonder of wonders, he was singing. The last time George had sung in the shower, Kim remembered, was on their anniversary three and a half years ago, just one day before things began to unravel. She rushed into the bathroom. "George! Are you all right?" Stepping out of the shower, her husband grinned at her. "I have never felt this good." He winked. "I think the medicine is kicking in." And with that he whisked her off her feet and into bed for a long-neglected session of lovemaking.

When everything comes together for the depressed person, feeling good can take him or her by surprise—and with that surprise, you, as caregiver are also thrown off. Though it's what you've longed for, it can be a shock to see a smile on a face that has frowned for so long, to hear a joke from someone who has consistently grumbled. For the depressed person it might be the first time he or she has ever felt so good.

Sometimes there is even a giddiness to the feeling—suddenly everything is beautiful and rich and worth celebrating. For a caregiver exhausted and spent after a rough ride through the illness, these changes may be a reason not for celebration, but rather for resentment and fear.

In your life together there is now a new normal. Now, this person whom you had to shepherd through the ins and outs of depression is functioning normally, is returning to work competently and contentedly, is playing with the kids and suggesting fun activities to try. Some of the things you learned to do to help you both cope are no longer needed, and you may be rebuffed when you slip into one of them out of habit. It takes a bit of time to adjust to this change.

When Ellen's partner Gladys came out of her depression, she was full of energy. Ellen, on the other hand, could only worry that she would be left behind in this new life of Gladys's, that there would be no room in her life for the tired and spent Ellen. When Ellen didn't react with enthusiasm to Gladys's suggestions for things like trips, nights out on the town, and new volunteer projects, she worried that Gladys would think her a killjoy. She was afraid Gladys would soon tire of suggesting new ideas that Ellen was too tired to execute, and would finally find that they didn't belong together at all.

Negative feelings are one of the many reactions to a depressed person's recovery. For a long time you've helped and guided and taken all the responsibility. With the depressed person's recovery, there is the feeling of being unneeded and therefore unappreciated and unwanted. The exhaustion from navigating the depression is a key reason for these feelings. Now you have no "job," now you are not needed, now you have to change your role.

We know in our minds, of course, that changing roles due to recovery is a positive step. It's getting used to the changes that takes patience and effort. For those in a marriage relationship or partnership, it means looking at each other as adults who have chosen to live together because they find that being together enhances both of their lives. For someone who has shepherded an elderly parent through depression, it means learning to look at each other as equal, capable adults again. For the parent whose child has recovered from depression, it is a matter of letting go of some of the fear, and appreciating the child's ability to grow and mature, safely and happily. For those who step out of postpartum depression, it is time to build bonds with the baby, laughing and singing and appreciating each other for weathering the rough times. Everyone in the situation has reason to celebrate now that the joyous dance of recovery has begun, though it can take time for caregivers to recuperate enough to recognize that fact.

"Anyone who says only sunshine brings happiness has never danced in the rain."

Unknown

Saying Goodbye to Old Patterns of Behavior

When recovery is in full force, we often find that the patterns of behavior we have slipped into persevere, long after they're no longer needed. Perhaps we were in the habit of waking our partner and getting him or her dressed and ready for the day, laying out his or her clothes, reminding him or her to brush his or her teeth, inspecting him or her before he or she left the house. Now, your partner is no longer burdened by the depression and is quite capable of managing a morning routine alone. It is hard to keep quiet and let them handle things for themselves, but it is necessary to their recovery that they be allowed to do so.

Allowing the depressed person to take on responsibility is necessary for your recovery as well. For a long time you have operated in a different mode, taking over as parent and caregiver, doing many of the things your depressed loved one could no longer do for him- or herself. Now you have to step back and allow your loved one to do these things alone. You have to "recover" from being a parent and caregiver.

One of the biggest helps in this recovery is for you to think before you speak. Chances are you were about to respond in a parent or caregiver role. Old habits are hard to break. Pausing and thinking allows you to reword what you were going to say or to decide against saying it at all. Such restraint will allow you and your loved one to regain some of the normal relationship you had before the depression began.

Try This

Wear a rubber band around your wrist, and each time you think of responding in the parent/caregiver role, snap the rubber band to remind yourself to stop and think. This simple action will help you become aware of the new behavior to which you are being called.

Sometimes, after recovery from depression, it can seem as if a relationship is starting again from square one. Both of you have to learn new ways of behaving and relating to each other. Keep the lines of communication open, and remember the "T" of PACT. Be truthful with your loved one about how you are feeling during this period of recovery. Let your loved one know if you are feeling left behind, feeling like you can't keep up. Spell out tasks you took on while your loved one was less able, and discuss openly what he or she is able to take on now. Be honest about how you felt about these tasks before and how you feel now. Ask him or her to be honest about how he or she feels about taking on more responsibility. Talk about ways in which you can both recover together. Acknowledge how difficult it is to lose the behavior patterns you moved into when you were the caregiver. When we are on the road of recovery, truth can make any relationship stronger, healthier, and full of dance.

Meditation

*"May your life be like a wildflower, growing
freely in the beauty and joy of each day."*

Native American Proverb

When we leave behind the darkness of depression and move into the light of recovery, we have to learn how to take in the light, how to let it warm us and remind us that we are loved. We need to become like wildflowers, growing freely into the beauty and joy of recovery, learning new behaviors, rediscovering our loved one, ready to rejoice in each new step each of us takes into the light. We might not always be ready to be that carefree wildflower. We might be afraid of the wind and of the insects that could attack us, but if we face the sun and throw our petals open to this new life, we will bloom. We will have come to know that life is good for both of us. We'll recognize that we are stronger for what we've encountered in the darkness. We can, with our loved

one, our community of support, and our Higher Power,
take on anything the light can bring us, including joy.

Lord, help me be open to the joy of recovery.

Learning to Enjoy Things Together Again

Recovery means we will be once again going back to things we might
have let go of during the dark time of depression. Perhaps it was shopping
together, going on dates, or seeing movies. Maybe it was a popcorn night
with games or a party with friends. Whatever good times we let go of during
depression, it is time to bring them back.

Talk together about things you want to bring back into your relationship.
If as parent and child you played board games together, revive that ritual,
making it a festive occasion. If you double-dated as roommates, try that
again. As always, though, talk with each other to monitor feelings and
fears and discuss things that you want to do differently this time around.
Remember that both of you are fragile. You are both recovering from illness
and both of you need the love and support from each other and your
supportive community.

Carl was finally seeing the goodness of life after the long bout of depression
he had suffered following the death of his wife. His daughter Emily was
by his side the entire time, seeing that he took his medicine, taking him
to doctor's appointments, and just seeing that he did something different
each day. Now that the medication was working, he felt great and he
wanted to revive their tradition of occasionally going out together on a
dad-and-daughter "date." But the last dinner that they'd had ended with
his walking out of the restaurant after severely berating the waitress and
the management and being rude to the other diners. He wasn't sure his
daughter would want to chance it again.

He and Emily sat down and talked about his concerns. Emily listened,
voicing some of her own concerns and fears. She felt that if they both

continued to talk honestly about their feelings, she didn't see what was wrong with trying it again. They agreed beforehand that if Carl felt at all uncomfortable or that anger was welling up in him, he would tap the table twice as a signal and suggest they leave. The two soon had dinner together and enjoyed each other's company very much. A much-valued activity was revived and enjoyed once again.

Communication during this time of recovery can't be stressed enough. A lot of hurtful things have happened during the time of depression, and healing takes time. Talking as Emily and Carl did is a step toward facing the fears and resuming activities you've missed.

Reflections

- *What activities would I like to resume that depression took from me and my loved one?*

- *What do I need to do to better communicate my thoughts and feelings to my loved one during this recovery period?*

- *What safeties can be put into place to ensure that both of us will be able to enjoy ourselves during the reviving of once-loved but long-forgotten activities?*

Fearing Depression Will Return

One of the biggest fears to surface during the time of recovery is fear of the return of depression. For many of us depression came as a surprise, and we are afraid it will surprise us again, right when we are feeling so good.

Yes, depression can return. It can broadside us again and again, but, as with anything in life, we can only do our best to be prepared and then ride out the storm whenever it comes. Medication has been known to stop working; circumstances might send us back into the darkness. Right now, though, our job is to enjoy recovery while keeping a watchful, but not intense, eye on how things are going for our loved one.

Don't overreact to situations you think might be a herald of the depression returning. Moodiness is just moodiness, not the ugly face of depression. Grouchiness is grouchiness, without the hint of anger returning. We have to acknowledge that we have been hurt by the depression of our loved one, and we may be fearful of the return of the darkness, so we may tend to overreact. Sometimes things are just what they are, with no agenda attached to them. You can still be alert to the signs of depression, but remember that these signs should be present for a sustained period of time, even weeks, before the diagnosis can be made. A one-time occurrence does not constitute depression.

Overreacting could create its own problems. When we are fearful, we can fall into old routines of behaving, perhaps taking back responsibilities that should rightly be our loved one's. We could set back recovery by creating insecurity in him or her. He or she might feel they're not improving, and fear that the depression is not gone. A fine balance must be achieved.

Talk together about how best to monitor the situation so overreaction doesn't occur and the good of recovery is not lost. In any relationship communication is key, and talking through recovery is important for all concerned so that a healthy, happy recovery is enjoyed by all.

Enjoying Recovery

During recovery, it is good to consider bringing PACT into play.

Go to your Higher Power and express thanks for this moment in time that allows you both to rejoice in each other's good health and happiness. Ask your Higher Power for the strength to be open to each other during the recovery so you can both grow stronger because of the depression.

Each day during recovery and beyond, find time to affirm each other, both for the courage it took to go through the depression and for the wonder and awe of a good recovery. Let each other know that you value each other and that your love is deep.

Draw on your community of support and have them celebrate recovery with you. Plan a party or a night of sharing to talk of the darkness and of the light, to remind each other of the importance of your support and care and love for each other.

Finally, keep that truth up and running. Be honest with your loved one and be honest with yourself. If you find your loved one or yourself slipping, talk about it, or act on it immediately, trusting that the truth will set you free to heal. Also, when appropriate, be truthful with sharing what you have gone through so that others might find hope and strength in your story.

Try This

There is a saying: "Do good, and don't get caught." Take some time today to do one little good thing for your loved one. Don't ask for credit or acclaim. You may be surprised at how much better this makes both of you feel. "Catch" your loved one in the act when he or she does something that especially pleases you, and let him or her know how it makes you feel. This kind of behavior builds on itself—it's self-rewarding and self-sustaining.

Dealing with depression is a journey on a long, hard road. For some of us, the journey isn't over; the darkness is still present. For others, the choice to end the journey has been made through divorce or estrangement or suicide. For some lucky individuals, the journey has taken us to recovery, where we can rejoice in all that is good and beautiful.

By dancing in the dark, both in the painful times and in the joyful times, we are able to affirm once again our humanness, our ability to love, and this truth: that you can dance anywhere, even if only in your heart.

Making the Tools Your Own

Though many in the medical profession suggest a combination of medication and therapy for treating depression, there is no "one-size-fits-all" way to survive the illness. Each depressed person must find his or her own unique path out of the darkness. The same holds true for those of us who suffer as we stand alongside, watching, coaching, encouraging. Though attention to self-care during this time is a necessity, each of us must find our own dance steps during this time of darkness.

It is our hope that among the various tools and suggestions in this book, you've found some that speak to you. In this appendix, we offer some ways for you to personalize these tools for your own use. (Use a separate notebook or journal where necessary.)

Stepping onto the Dance Floor

Quotes That Spoke to Me

In your notebook, make note of the quotes in this book or elsewhere that made you pause, gave you inspiration, or in some way touched you.

Square-Dancing with PACT

Use this space to write, to make a list, or to draw what's going on during this time.

PRAYER

Here's my list of my spiritual needs at this time:

Some thoughts to help me keep in touch with my Higher Power:

New ways for me to pray:

Thoughts, emotions, or whatever I want to share with my Higher Power:

In what ways am I turning to my Higher Power for moments of quiet?

AFFIRMATION

List everything I've ever heard anyone say about me that is good and affirming:

What unique qualities do I possess that can be valuable in this difficult situation?

Who can I look to in order to receive affirmation right now? What affirmation would be healing for me?

COMMUNITY

List names of people I can be with just to have fun and get away from depression:

List names of people who can assist me when I need a break:

Who can help me with appointments, daily tasks, check-ins, etc.?

What are my thoughts and feelings about community?

TRUTH
Here are the people I can trust with the truth about my situation:

When do I avoid the truth, and when do I embrace it?

What are my thoughts and feelings about truth?

My Dance Card: My Plan for Self-Care
List anything I can do to take care of myself during this difficult time:

Who can help me with my self-care?

What prevents me from taking care of myself?

What would I most like to do in taking care of myself?

Dancing Out of the Dark and into the Light

Hip-hop
What brings me joy? List as many things as possible, from simple things to huge things, that make me smile and fill me with a sense of joy:

How can I experience these things even in this time of darkness?

Slow Dance
In what ways am I turning to my Higher Power for moments of quiet, peace, or centering?

Recall times I have felt the presence of my Higher Power:

Twist
What is creating frustration for me at the present time?

How can I remedy the frustration I'm feeling?

Tango
In what ways are my loved one and I going in different directions?

How can that change?

In what ways have we drawn closer?

Line Dance
How do I feel when my loved one and I are in sync?

How can I let him or her know what that means to me?

Square Dance
How does allowing a community of support to take part in my dance make me feel?

What might be the outcomes of turning to a community of support?

Jitterbug
When things are frantic with me and my loved one, how does that make me feel?

What do I find most effective in reducing stress and creating calm?

Waltz
What do I most appreciate on the days my loved one and I glide along smoothly?

If I am in recovery with my loved one, what feelings crop up in me?

Polka
What's the best part of celebrating with my loved one?

What is happening in my life right now that is a reason to kick up my heels and dance?

How can I keep dancing no matter what depression has done to my life and my relationships?

Also available from Central Recovery Press

www.centralrecoverypress.com

Pain Recovery

A Day without Pain (Revised and Updated)
Mel Pohl, MD, FASAM
ISBN-10: 1-936290-62-6
ISBN-13: 978-1-936290-62-8
$15.95 US

Pain Recovery: How to Find Balance and
Reduce Suffering from Chronic Pain
Mel Pohl, MD, FASAM; Frank J. Szabo, Jr., LADC; Dan Shiode, PhD;
Rob Hunter, PhD
ISBN-10: 0-9799869-9-0
ISBN-13: 978-0-9799869-9-4
$20.95 US

Pain Recovery for Families: How to Find Balance When
Someone Else's Chronic Pain Becomes Your Problem Too
Mel Pohl, MD, FASAM; Frank J. Szabo, Jr., LADC; Dan Shiode, PhD;
Rob Hunter, PhD
ISBN-10: 0-9818482-3-0
ISBN-13: 978-0-9818482-3-5
$20.95 US

Meditations for Pain Recovery
Tony Greco
ISBN-10: 0-9819482-8-1
ISBN-13: 978-0-9818482-8-0
$16.95 US

Inspirational

The Truth Begins with You: Reflections to Heal Your Spirit
Claudia Black, PhD
ISBN-10: 1-936290-61-8
ISBN-13: 978-1-936290-61-1
$17.95 US

Above and Beyond: 365 Meditations for
Transcending Chronic Pain and Illness
J. S. Dorian
ISBN-10: 1-936290-66-9
ISBN-13: 978-1-936290-66-6
$15.95 US

Guide Me in My Recovery: Prayers for
Times of Joy and Times of Trial
Rev. John T. Farrell, PhD
ISBN-10: 1-936290-00-6
ISBN-13: 978-1-936290-00-0
$12.95 US

Special hardcover gift edition:
ISBN-10: 1-936290-02-2
ISBN-13: 978-1-936290-02-4
$19.95 US

The Soul Workout: Getting and Staying Spiritually Fit
Helen H. Moore
ISBN-10: 0-9799869-8-2
ISBN-13: 978-0-9799869-8-7
$12.95 US

Becoming Normal: An Ever-Changing Perspective
Mark Edick
ISBN-10: 0-9818482-1-4
ISBN-13: 978-0-9818482-1-1
$14.95 US

Dopefiend: A Father's Journey from Addiction to Redemption
Tim Elhajj
ISBN-10: 1-936290-63-4
ISBN-13: 978-1-936290-63-5
$16.95 US

Advocacy

Picking Up the Pieces without Picking Up: A Guidebook Through Victimization for People in Recovery
Jennifer Storm
ISBN-10: 1-936290-64-2
ISBN-13: 978-1-936290-64-2
$15.95 US

Young Adult and Young Reader

First Star I See
Jaye Andras Caffrey, illustrated by Lynne Adamson
ISBN-10: 1-936290-01-4
ISBN-13: 978-1-936290-01-7
$12.95 US

Tails of Recovery: Addicts and the Pets That Love Them
Nancy A. Schenck
ISBN-10: 0-9799869-6-6
ISBN-13: 978-0-9799869-6-3
$19.95 US

Of Character: Building Assets in Recovery
Denise D. Crosson, PhD
ISBN-10: 0-9799869-2-3
ISBN-13: 978-0-9799869-2-5
$12.95 US

Memoirs

Riding a Straight and Twisty Road: Motorcycles,
Fellowship, and Personal Journeys
James Hesketh
ISBN-10: 1-936290-05-7
ISBN-13: 978-1-936290-05-5
$16.95 US

Leave the Light On: A Memoir of Recovery and Self-Discovery
Jennifer Storm
ISBN-10: 0-9818482-2-2
ISBN-13: 978-0-9818482-2-8
$14.95 US

The Mindful Addict: A Memoir of the Awakening of a Spirit
Tom Catton
ISBN-10: 0-9818482-7-3
ISBN-13: 978-0-9818482-7-3
$18.95 US

The Secret of Willow Ridge: Gabe's Dad Finds Recovery
Helen H. Moore, illustrated by John Blackford
Foreword by Claudia Black, PhD
ISBN-10: 0-9818482-0-6
ISBN-13: 978-0-9818482-0-4
$12.95 US

Mommy's Gone to Treatment
Denise D. Crosson, PhD, illustrated by Mike Motz
ISBN-10: 0-9799869-1-5
ISBN-13: 978-0-9799869-1-8
$14.95 US

Mommy's Coming Home from Treatment
Denise D. Crosson, PhD, illustrated by Mike Motz
ISBN-10: 0-9799869-4-X
ISBN-13: 978-0-9799869-4-9
$14.95 US

Relationships

From Heartbreak to Heart's Desire: Developing a Healthy GPS (Guy Picking System)
Dawn Maslar, MS
ISBN-10: 0-9818482-6-5
ISBN-13: 978-0-9818482-6-6
$14.95 US

Disentangle: When You've Lost Your Self in Someone Else
Nancy L. Johnston, MS, LPC, LSATP
ISBN-10: 1-936290-03-0
ISBN-13: 978-1-936290-03-1
$15.95 US

A Spiritual Path to a Healthy Relationship: A Practical Approach
Steve McCord, MFT, and Angie McCord, CC
ISBN-10: 1-9362-9065-0
ISBN-13: 978-1-9362-9065-9
$15.95 US

Journals and Reference

My First Year in Recovery: A Journal for the Journey (Second Edition)
The Editors of Central Recovery Press
ISBN-10: 0-9818482-4-9
ISBN-13: 978-0-9818482-4-2
$19.95 US

My Five-Year Recovery Planner: Looking to
the Future, One Day at a Time
The Editors of Central Recovery Press
ISBN-10: 0-9818482-9-X
ISBN-13: 978-0-9818482-9-7
$19.95 US

My Pain Recovery Journal
The Editors of Central Recovery Press
ISBN-10: 0-9799869-7-4
ISBN-13: 978-0-9799869-7-0
$17.95 US

Recovery A to Z: A Handbook of Twelve-Step Key
Terms and Phrases (Revised and Updated)
The Editors of Central Recovery Press
ISBN-10: 1-936290-04-9
ISBN-13: 978-1-936290-04-8
$15.95 US